30 Ways to Survive Dining Hall and Dorm Room Food:

Tips to Avoid the Freshman 15

Penelope M. Klatell, PhD, RN

Table of Contents

Introduction

College: So many changes—it seems like everything is new and different and it happens all at once. But there's a constant—something that stays the same: food and your need to eat. But are you gearing up to eat and drink anything you want, at any time that you choose—just because you can (and because Mom isn't there to say no)?

Your body's need for food might stay the same, but your eating patterns certainly won't be. The structure of your day will be entirely different, so when, where, with whom, and what do you eat?

Freshman 15, an expression commonly used in the US (other countries have their own names), refers to the weight college students often gain during their freshman year.

There are many possible reasons for this weight gain and almost all of them involve a change in eating patterns and food choices. Fatty and carbohydrate-rich food; dorm life; food availability in dining halls, student centers, and campus stores; close to campus fast-food places;

all-nighters; alcohol; a change in activity patterns; the party life; and no more scrutiny by Mom and Dad all have their own effect on what you eat, where you eat, and why you eat.

The "15" in Freshman 15 is an arbitrary number. A study showed that college freshmen gain (eatouteatwell.com/freshman weight gain) between 2.5 to 3.5 pounds, on average, over the course of their first year of college. The amount varies, but many students say that weight gain doesn't stop—it continues throughout and after college (eatouteatwell.com/college weight), with women gaining, on average, seven to nine pounds and men between 12 and 13 pounds during college and another 1.5 pounds a year in the first four years after college.

The Solution

The most workable solution is to prevent weight gain—the dreaded freshman 15 (or whatever your number might be). It's not so difficult to do: it's all about making informed choices and recognizing that sometimes the best choice to be made in any given situation is not necessarily perfect but the best one for the situation that you're in.

Make the best choice for you wherever you are: but be smart about it.

How To Use This Book

Use this book for tips and as a reference. Each chapter is short and about one subject and includes suggestions for actions that you can take. There may be occasional duplication of some information but that is intentional and designed to help you get your questions answered in each specific chapter.

1.

What's In Your Mini-Fridge And In The Boxes Under Your Bed?

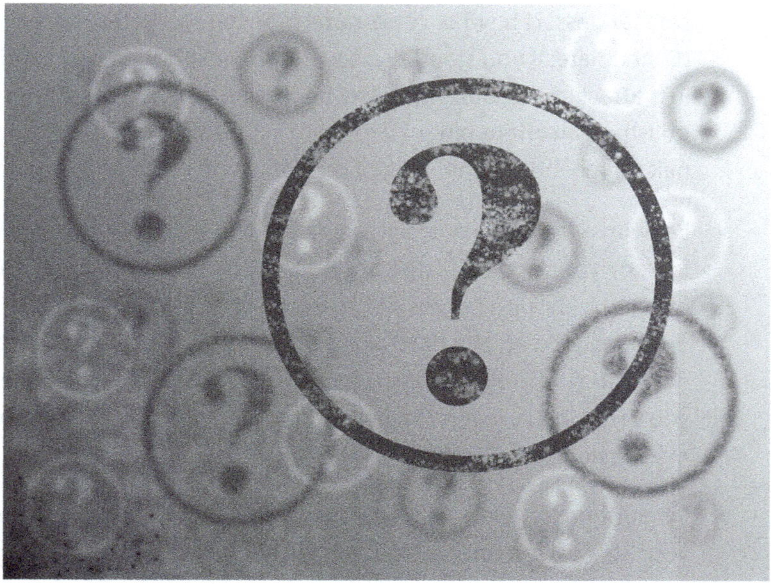

Freedom. You're away from home. There are no parents looking over your shoulder. You can eat anything you want any time that you want.

There's food around in quantities that you're not used to. One sight of open bags of chips, cookies, and pretzels and the notion of sweet/salty/fatty/caloric food has embedded itself in your brain and has firmly taken root.

What To Do

The food is there. It's part of dorm life. Just figure out what works best for you so you can monitor portions and avoid eating the stuff that makes you feel groggy and foggy. How healthy the food is might not be foremost in your mind, but for the sake of your health at least pay some attention to what you're putting into your body.

Some Tips:

- Use a plate. Always put your food on a plate or in a bowl—the smaller the better. The size of the plate—or bowl—or container can often determine how much you ultimately eat. Make it a smaller dessert bowl or plate, not a monster size cereal bowl or dinner plate. If you stand there with fork or spoon in hand and just attack the container, in the blink of an eye it's possible to polish off an entire pint of ice cream, a double piece of cake or half (or maybe a whole) bag of cookies.

- Eat with a teaspoon or small fork not with a tablespoon, a large fork, or your fingers. Large amounts of food disappear much more quickly with fingers or large utensils as shovels. The food disappears down the hatch so quickly that your brain doesn't have time to register that you've eaten something—until you've probably overeaten way too much food and way too many calories.

- Don't bring leftovers back to your room. Don't let them invade your space. Don't bring back the leftover pizza or the leftover cake from the party, either.

- Hide the stuff that tempts you. Out of sight, out of mind is really true. We all tend to eat more when it's right in front of us. Food we like—especially higher calorie sugary, fatty, and salty foods—trigger cravings and eating.

- Care packages can be a bonus or a problem. Talk to your parents about what you need and want. Come to an agreement about food with your roommate(s), too.

2.

Do The Words "Cafeteria Style" And "All You Can Eat" Send Your Inner Calorie Counter Into Panic Mode?

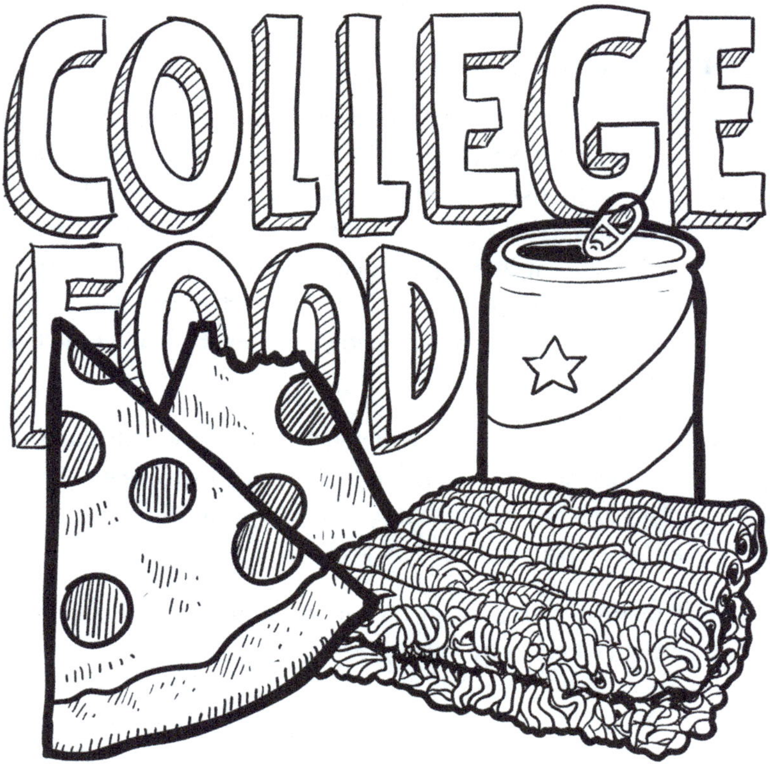

Are you challenged by the incredible array of dining hall food just begging to be heaped on your plate? How do you decide what to choose and how much to take when the amount of food is massive, filled with variety—and no one is looking over your shoulder reminding you of what to eat—or not to eat.

You've Got To Have Some Kind Of Game Plan

Having a general eating game plan will help you with your food choices and also with your portion sizes.

Some people choose to have certain food on certain days: chicken on Tuesdays, pasta on Friday, salad for lunch on Wednesdays on so on. Others stick to one type of choice: from the grill versus pasta.

The bottom line is that you're in control of what you put into your body. The choice is yours.

What To Do

- We often eat with our eyes—if we see something delicious, we want to eat it. So, don't look at it. Keep your back to the food table or choose to sit where you can't see the food display—preferably a seat that's some distance away. How long can you sit and stare at cheesy pizza or mounds of fried chicken without wanting to sample? Not having the food in your line of sight helps to keep your mind—and your stomach—off of the food choices.

- Choose a smaller plate and you'll eat less. Try switching from a dinner plate to a salad plate. Research (eatouteatwell.com/plate size) has shown that by switching to a 10-inch plate from a 12-inch plate you eat 22% less.

- Engage in conversation. It's hard to keep shoving food in your mouth when you're talking.

- Nibbling while you're filling your plate really tacks on calories. Bites of bread crusts, a piece of bacon, and French fries are small and easy to forget. Make up your mind not to sample before you sit down to eat and stick to your plan or you'll have shoved down a thousand calories before you know it.

- What are you putting on your plate? Why sacrifice your calories for something that you don't like? Of course, don't eliminate whole food groups. Even for vegetable haters there's got to be a few vegetables you'll eat.

- Distance helps. Sit at the periphery of the dining hall. Having to get up and walk past lots people—many of whom you know—while balancing a plate filled to the brim can serve as a "seconds" and "thirds" deterrent.

- Before putting any food on your plate, just cruise the food stations to eyeball all of the choices. Decide what's going to energize you and not mess too badly with the calorie range that you want to maintain.

- Make up your mind what you're going to have, put it on your plate, sit down with your back to the food displays, and enjoy what you've decided to eat.

- Avoid seconds and picking food off of a plate that someone has generously piled high with a selection of cookies and brownies and put in the middle of the table for everyone to share (if you can, shove that plate out of arms' reach).

- If you decide you really will feel totally deprived if you don't indulge in one of those delicious baked goods, choose one without loads of thick buttery crumbs on top, cut it in half or in thirds and be satisfied with that amount. Put it on a separate small plate that you can easily push away from you. Keeping it on your main plate or even a smaller one that's easily reachable means you'll be nibbling away at it the entire time.

What's Your Food Choice And Why: Some Questions To Ask Yourself

A quick checklist of questions:

- What's my tried and true meal that can be my fallback or my "go to" meal for breakfast, lunch, or dinner? What type of food did I grow up with? Did that type of food give me energy, strength, and clarity?

- How do certain kinds of food make me feel? Do I feel like garbage after eating red meat or drinking a glass of milk? Stay away from foods that don't make you feel good. Just because someone else eats them doesn't mean you have to. Ditto for alcoholic beverages. If drinking makes you feel lousy you don't have to do it because others are (disclaimer: most freshmen are under the legal drinking age and this should not be taken as an endorsement to drink or purchase alcoholic beverages).

- Is it delicious? Why waste calories on something that doesn't taste good or has little or no nutritional value. But there are two sides to this coin. Just because something is good for you doesn't mean that it has to taste bad. On the flip side—maybe you don't like a certain food even if it's a nutritional superstar. There are lots of delicious and healthy foods so why force yourself to eat what you don't like? Just try to balance your food choices and pick something else from the colorful rainbow of foods.

- If I eat this, how am I going to feel half an hour or an hour from now? When you eat a big bowl of pasta at lunch do you have to prop your head up on a book to try to stay awake? Learn to identify the relationship between certain foods and how your body physically and emotionally reacts to them. Do some make you sleepy, crabby, alert, or give you energy?

- Is this the right portion size for me? Portion control is essential for weight management. Learn to eyeball portion sizes and commit to a personal "no seconds" policy at least 80% of the time (nobody is—or should be—perfect).

- Do I really want to eat this or am I doing it just because . . . (you supply the answer—some typical ones are: everyone else is eating it, or it's fried chicken day, or "I had a tough day, I deserve it").

3.

How To Use Food To Keep Off The Energy Roller Coaster

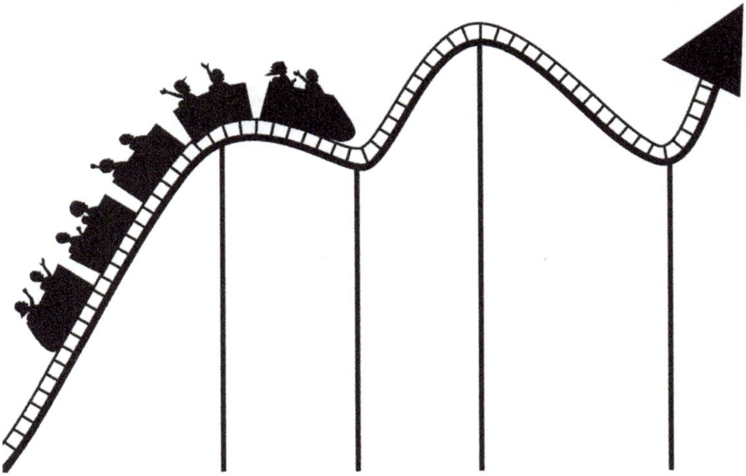

Does this sound like your day?

- You drag yourself out of bed grumpy and fuzzy
- A large coffee and muffin or donut perks you up
- Around 10:30 you grab another donut or a protein bar when you start to drag
- 3PM and you're having trouble keeping your eyes open
- After dinner, snacks in hand, you settle down to write a paper and doze off over the computer.

Hippocrates Would Have Said, "I've Got A Solution"

Almost 2,500 years ago Hippocrates, the father of medicine, famously said: "Let food be thy medicine and medicine be thy food."

Hippocrates' line of thinking—and current scientific research --support the fact that food is both the culprit and the treatment for a big part of our lack of energy, muddled thinking, and mid-afternoon drowsy eyes.

What Food Does For Your Body

Food is your body's fuel—it's the gas in your tank that gives your body the energy it needs to function. Your cell phone needs to be charged, your car needs gas, and your body needs food.

Food boosts your energy by giving your body the calories and fluid it needs to function and it stokes your metabolism so that it works efficiently.

The type of food you eat affects your metabolism and your brain chemistry—which then affects your energy level and your mood. When and how frequently you eat plays a big role in your energy levels throughout the day.

Your body has the easiest time digesting carbohydrates (starches, sugars and dietary fiber). It turns them into glucose, the body's preferred fuel. Glucose is the sugar that travels in your bloodstream, and the only fuel normally used by brain cells. Because the neurons in your brain can't store glucose, they need your bloodstream to deliver a steady supply.

Why Carbs Are Important: A Simple And Complex Answer

Simple carbs, often called "simple sugars,"—table sugar, syrups, and most sugars found in refined and processed foods and drinks, break down easily, quickly raise your blood sugar levels, and give you a short-lived boost.

Sugary food causes your pancreas to secrete insulin, which triggers your cells to get the excess glucose out of your bloodstream. That means there's less glucose available to your brain and neurons. Because they can't store glucose, they end up with an energy crisis—leaving you struggling to concentrate and feeling spaced-out, weak, confused, and irritable.

The Slower Burn

Because complex carbs—like the ones in whole grains, beans, and vegetables—take longer to breakdown, your body digests them more slowly and they supply energy at a slower and more sustained rate.

Fruit and dairy contain simple but nutrient-rich carbs. The fiber in whole fruit helps to slow down digestion but fruit juice, soda and other sugary drinks lack fiber and are filled with rapidly digested simple sugar. Dairy gets its energy sustaining power from the combination of its simple carb, lactose, along with fat and protein.

Healthy Fats Can Be Energizing

After carbs, fats are a big source of energy. Feed your body healthy fats from foods like avocados, olives, fatty fish, seeds, nuts, and vegetable and nut oils. A healthy energizing snack with good fats might be one ounce (14 halves) of walnuts or other nuts, which also contain some protein and complex carbs.

Protein For A Longer Lasting Energy Boost

Because of the time it takes to break down its amino acids, protein also supplies longer-lasting energy. Prime protein sources are poultry, lean meat, certain types of dairy, fish, eggs, beans, nuts, and lentils.

Many protein-rich foods have other energy-boosting benefits, too. Poultry, red meat, fish, eggs, beans, nuts and seeds contain iron and B vitamins. Iron helps to transport oxygen to your organs—which helps with fatigue. B vitamins help release energy. To prevent energy crashes try combining a low-fat protein with a complex carbohydrate, like turkey or grilled chicken on whole wheat bread or pita.

Keep A Full Tank

To keep off of that energy roller coaster you need to eat the right food at the right time. Skipping meals isn't a good idea. Your body needs fuel, preferably high-octane fuel, just like a performance car. If you don't give it the right gas it certainly has trouble running smoothly.

Start the day off right. If you want to boost your energy and mood, don't skip breakfast. The best breakfasts have plenty of fiber, nutrients from whole-grain carbs, good fats, and some type of lean protein. Try some low fat Greek yogurt with fruit and a sprinkling of whole grain cereal.

Energy sustaining snacks can be peanut butter or low-fat cheese with whole grain crackers, veggies with hummus, whole-grain cereal with milk, or a small portion of nuts with some fruit. Be prepared and carry some snacks with you so you don't go for a long time without fuel. Stash some in your backpack or dorm room so the good stuff is always readily available and the allure of the vending machine isn't so great.

Don't Hover On Empty

Don't let your tank get empty—you'll end up eating everything in sight, starting with simple carbs. To keep your blood sugar stable and to have well fed brain cells have something to eat (a meal or a snack) every three to four hours. Meals or snacks made of complex carbohydrates, protein, a small amount of healthy fat, and accompanied by something to drink (preferably water) provide the type of fuel your body needs to stay off of the energy roller coaster.

4.

You Probably Should Eat A Healthy Breakfast: Here's Why

You're not in high school any more. There's no one on your case about eating a good breakfast before you go to class.

Why You Should Eat Breakfast

Do you want to stay awake, concentrate, and get stuff done? Breakfast can help—and there are all kinds, some far better for long-lasting fuel than others.

There are "grab and go" breakfasts and there are "sit down in the dining hall" breakfasts. There are cinnamon rolls with icing, pop tarts, oatmeal, eggs, bagels, and protein bars. They're all not created equal—breakfast should contain protein and fiber if you're aiming for clear-headed thinking, energy, and a stomach that doesn't start growling in the middle of class.

The advice to eat a good breakfast has been around for centuries. It's clear how it affects your body's biology, but now it's been documented that eating a healthy breakfast—especially one high in protein—can leave you feeling fuller, less hungry throughout the day, and help your attention span and memory.

Researchers studied groups of teens who either skipped breakfast, ate a 500 calorie breakfast of cereal and milk with normal amounts of protein, or a higher protein meal. Eating breakfast made people feel fuller and not as hungry during the morning.

The conclusion: eating breakfast—especially one rich in protein—might be a good strategy to help control your appetite and to prevent overeating.

So What Should You Eat For Breakfast?

Breakfast doesn't have to be fancy, it doesn't have to be huge, and you don't have to sit at a table to eat it.

If you make it to the dining hall for breakfast, there's a whole range of good choices.

- Eggs are loaded with protein and won't weigh you down. Bacon and sausage are protein heavy but are salty and have preservatives.

- Oatmeal has good long-staying fiber as do many –but not all—cereals. Some cereals are loaded with sugar. Huge bowls and cereal dispensers that just keep dropping cereal into them are way too tempting and can dispense three or four servings at a pop (actual suggested serving sizes of cereal can be quite small). Add milk to cereal or oatmeal for some protein and some fruit for some sweet nutrition.

- Grab a container of low-fat yogurt and top it with some cereal or fruit. A banana, raisins, and other dried fruit work well as do small, prepackaged containers of sliced peaches and pears or applesauce.

- Stuff a pita or whole grain tortilla with refried beans or sun-dried tomatoes and a slice of cheese and warm it up in a microwave.

- Keep a stash of apples, bananas, and oranges on hand. Pair them with some cheese sticks and/or a handful of nuts. Awesome, easy, and filling.

- PB & J doesn't have to be lunch food. Put some on crackers or whole grain bread. Travels well. Not a fan of peanut butter? Try sunflower or almond butter. Nuts and seeds added to yogurt or cereal—or just by the handful—are great nutritional sources.

- There are a ton of protein bars and protein drinks out there. Some are pretty good—some are pretty bad. Look for ones with a higher protein count (aim for 15 grams per serving), fiber, low sugar and minimal preservatives. The ultimate grab and go breakfast or mid-morning snack.

- Smoothies can be great—or can be loaded with sugar. Just check that they have some protein added from yogurt or whey protein powder.

- Don't underestimate the value of a low fat latte or hot chocolate made with low-fat milk. Protein, hot, and good tasting!

- Remember to keep your body hydrated with water!

5.

Is Your Coffee Giving You A Muffin Top?

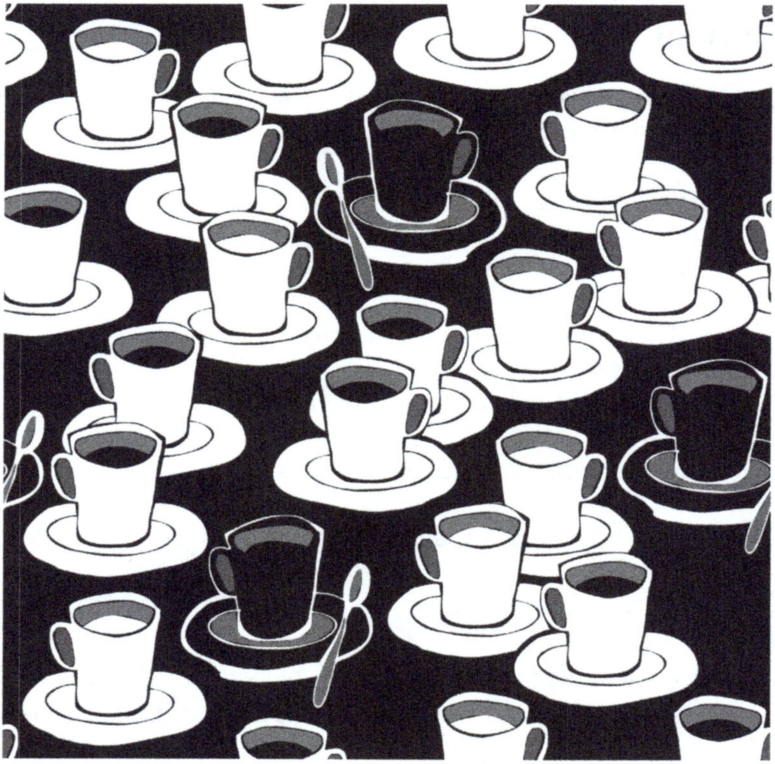

Morning coffee. Mid-afternoon. 3AM—when you're struggling with a paper. Hot, cold, it doesn't really matter. How do you like your coffee? Black, light and sweet, regular?

As you dump sugar and pour cream into mugs, thermoses, and those too hot to touch cardboard take-out containers, have you ever thought about how many calories you're actually adding to an otherwise very low calorie drink? Probably not. They're calories not usually measured and all too easy to forget.

What Do You Put Into Your Coffee Or Tea?

How much milk or half and half do you add to your coffee or tea? How much sugar? Bet you don't have a clue. We all do a freehand pour. Try measuring how much you actually pour into your cup and you might be really surprised.

The Facts:

- Black brewed coffee (and tea) has around two calories in an eight-ounce cup. Not a bad deal.
- Heavy cream, 1 tablespoon: 52 calories
- Half-and-half, 1 tablespoon: 20 calories
- Whole milk, 1 tablespoon: 9 calories
- 2% (low fat) milk; 1 tablespoon: 7 calories
- Non-fat milk, 1 tablespoon: 5 calories
- Table sugar, 1 tablespoon: 49 calories; 1 teaspoon: 16 calories

Wow—It Can Add Up

Say you have three grande (Starbucks)—or large (Dunkin' Donuts)—coffees a day. Each is 20 ounces or 2.5 times the size of a traditional 8 ounce cup.

If you add 4 tablespoons of half and half and three teaspoons of sugar to each—which sounds like a lot but is very east to do—that's 128 calories for what you add and around 5 calories for the coffee for a total of 133 calories for each grande/large cup of coffee

If you have three of those daily that's 399 calories a day or the equivalent of 145,635 calories a year.

In Case You're Tempted By Something More

Here's more nutritional info for Starbucks and Dunkin' Donuts drinks (similar coffee drinks served by other coffee chains will have around the same nutrition for the same size cup):

- Starbucks Caffe Latte, grande (16 ounces), 2% milk: 190 calories, 7g fat, 18g carbs, 12g protein
- Starbucks Cappuchino, grande (16 ounces), 2% milk: 120 calories, 4g fat, 12g carbs, 8g protein
- Starbucks Peppermint White Chocolate Mocha, grande (16 ounces), 2% milk, no whipped cream: 440 calories, 10g fat, 75g carbs, 13g protein
- Starbucks Hot Chocolate, grande (16 ounces), 2% milk with whipped cream: 370 calories, 16g fat, 50g carbs, 14g protein, 25mg caffeine. Without whipped cream: 290 calories
- Dunkin' Donuts Mint Hot Chocolate, medium: 310 calories, 10g fat, 52g carbs, 2g protein
- Dunkin' Donuts Vanilla Chai: 330 calories, 8g fat, 53g carbs, 11g protein

6.

Did You Eat Too Much? Blame Your Buddies At The Table

How many people do you routinely sit with in the dining hall? Not all the people surrounding you, but the number of friends at your table. Amazingly, how many people you eat with can make a big difference in how much you end up eating. If you have eight at your table you might end up eating 96% more than if you ate alone!

That's not to say that you should limit the number of friends you eat with—it should just make you aware that friends, unintentionally, can influence how much and how fast you eat.

Most of us tend to stay at the table longer when we're with others. The longer you're at the table, the more you'll eat. Maybe it's due to mindlessly nibbling while someone else talks, the manners you learned in fifth grade, or because you're just having fun and enjoying your food.

You tend to mimic the people at your table, too. It's almost as though how much you eat and how fast you eat is contagious. If your friends eat fast, you eat fast. If they eat a lot, you eat a lot. Have you ever seen families walking down the street and the proportionate body size of the family group tends to be similar?

How Much More Do You Eat When Others Are At The Table?

Compared to eating alone you eat, on average:

- 35% more if you eat with one other person

- 75% more with four at the table
- 96% more with a group of seven or more

One reason this happens is a phenomenon called "social facilitation" (eatouteatwell.com/social facilitation), or the actions that are stimulated by the sight and sound of other people doing the same thing that you're doing. When you're eating in groups social facilitation helps override your brain's signals that tell you you're full and satisfied—which allows you to eat more even when you're not hungry.

What Can You Do?

- Don't isolate yourself. Sharing meals with others is really important, but you can give some thought to how many people you're eating with, who they are, and why you're sitting with them.
- If you want to have a blast and don't care about how much you eat—eat with a big group and chow down. If you want sushi and they're a burger and ribs crowd, you might want to think twice.
- If you want to be careful about what and how much you eat, have lunch with your salad (dressing on the side, please) friends rather than the pepperoni pizza group.
- Have in mind what you want to order ahead of time so you don't end up going with the flow and ordering what everyone else is having.
- Know your "safe meals." Learn what the calories and contents are of a few meals that are common to the restaurants you frequent. If you're stuck, or don't know what a menu entrée really contains, always order grilled chicken or fish with a side salad and/or vegetable.
- Since you tend to adjust your eating pace to that of your companions, sit next to the slow eaters rather than the speed eaters if you're trying to control how much goes into your mouth.

7.

Mindless Bites Pack On The Pounds

When you start having trouble getting your jeans to easily snap, give some thought to your "mindless bites"—those "shove it in your mouth without thinking about it" bites of food.

Have you ever:

- Snagged some candy from a friend's stash
- Licked cookie dough off the beaters
- Finished the crust off of someone else's grilled cheese or pizza
- Eaten handfuls of goldfish from an open bowl
- Liberally sampled the free "want to try" foods in the market?

We're on food decision overload a good part of the time—which helps to explain why we forget some of the food we pop into our mouths (we also forget because we want to ignore the calories, too)!

The Weighty Problem

Here's the "weighty" problem. Each of those mindless bites (eatouteatwell.com/mindlessbites)—those food choices that are part of the 200+ food decisions (eatouteatwell.com/food decisions) we make every day can add up to—on average—25 calories (sometimes more, sometimes less). There are quite a few mindless bites in half a large cookie or the broken pieces in the bottom of a bag of chips.

Because they're mindless, you forget about them and their calories. They're such quick pops into your mouth, you don't even have a chance to really taste them and it probably doesn't even register in your brain that you've eaten some food.

Here are some startling numbers: four mindless bites a day at about 25 calories apiece (above and beyond your daily calorie needs) means possibly gaining slightly less than a pound a month (it takes extra 3500 calories to gain a pound and 100 extra calories a day x 30 days = 3,000 calories). Ouch!

What To Do

Be aware of what you're eating—especially when you're not really eating a meal. Start keeping track of when and where you're most likely to indulge in mindless bites. You'd be surprised at how much you can mindlessly eat while you're walking, talking, socializing, working, watching games, and driving.

Try writing down what you eat for a few days—as soon as you eat it—either the old fashioned way or with one of the many apps. A written or online record is hard to refute. It's an amazing accountability check—and a very "in your face" account of how much you're truly eating because, honestly, do you really know?

8.

Why Do You Eat More Even When You're Stuffed?

You've been eating all day. Eating everything—a bagel for breakfast, a cinnamon bun for a midmorning snack, lunch in the dining hall, soda and a cupcake in the afternoon, fried chicken for dinner, and a 9PM trip to the vending machine.

Somehow There's Room For More Food

Amazingly, the signal to stop eating isn't usually because your stomach is full (except in some extreme cases), but a combination of things: what you taste, chew, swallow; how much you think about the food you are eating; and the length of time it takes you to eat.

The faster most people eat, the more they eat. Eating quickly doesn't give your brain the chance to get the message that you're not hungry any more. It takes up to 20 minutes for your body and brain to get the message—a satiation signal—and realize that you're full. Think about how much you can eat in that time span of 20 minutes—a burger, fries, pie, pizza, ice cream—and that's all in bonus time: the time after your stomach is full but your brain hasn't gotten the message yet.

What To Do

- Slow down when you eat. Give your brain a chance to catch up. How many times have you chowed down at lunch and then, almost immediately, decided that you're still hungry? So, you eat a whole bunch more—once again in a short period of time. Then, about half an hour later your belly feels like it's going to explode.

- Slower eating, more chewing, and better pacing gives your brain a chance to sync its signals with the messages generated from putting food in your stomach.
- Get up and do something else and promise yourself if you're still hungry in 20 minutes you can have more. In most cases, after the 20 or so minutes, your belly and brain will both be happy and you won't want more to eat.

9.

Traffic-Light Food Choices: Red (Once In A While), Yellow (Maybe Yes, Maybe No), And Green (Probably A Good Choice)

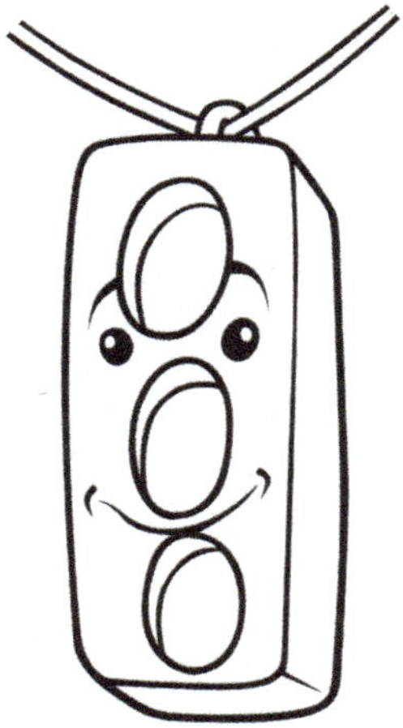

You can eat really well and save a whole lot of not-so-good for you calories by look for keywords that can clue you into extra fat, sugar, and calories.

Food descriptions, whether they're on a menu or on a sign on the wall in the cafeteria or deli, are filled with descriptive and sometimes mouth-watering words. They're meant to:

- entice you to pick certain items by making them sound scrumptious
- make you think that a food, sauce, or dressing is lower in calories or an awesome health food

Key Words To Look For

Here are some tips for recognizing the menu words and descriptions that can help you make your best caloric choices (of course, portion size plays a big role, too).

A menu item will have extra calories if it is:

- smothered in sauce
- covered or layered with cheese
- loaded with butter, oil, cream, mayonnaise, or dressing
- "sugared-up" even if it doesn't taste sweet
- made from a fatty cut of meat
- made with hidden sugar or flour and/or some type of fat for thickening
- described as big, huge, or all you can eat

Green Light (Probably A Good Choice) words or phrases:

- Barbequed
- Blanched
- Boiled
- Fat free
- Garden fresh
- Grilled/Broiled/Charbroiled/Seared
- Poached
- Primavera
- Red sauce/ Marinara

- Roasted
- Seasoned/Spiced/Rubbed
- Steamed

Quick hint: Words ending in the letter "d" are frequently on the okay list, for instance: poached, boiled, grilled, and steamed. Some notable exceptions are: fried, and the "b-d" words: buttered, battered, and breaded.

Yellow Light "Caution" (Maybe Yes, Maybe No) words or phrases:

These are words frequently used on menus to describe "yellow light foods,"—foods that should be chosen cautiously because they may or may not be healthy choices.

- Almandine/Almondine
- Baked
- Basted
- Glazed
- High Fiber
- Honey-dipped
- Light/Lite
- Marinated
- Panini
- Reduced
- Seasoned
- Stewed
- Stir-Fried/Sauteed
- Vegetarian
- Vinaigrette

Red Light (Once In A While) words and phrases:

Really think hard before eating food described with these words and phrases:

- Au gratin/Cheesy/Parmigiana
- Aioli
- Alfredo
- Battered/Encrusted/Crusted
- Bearnaise/Hollandaise
- Bet you can't finish it/ Bottomless/Value/Giant/Jumbo/Loaded
- Bisque
- Breaded
- Buttery / Buttered
- Carbonara
- Casserole
- Cheesy/Gooey/Melted
- Chicken fried/Pan fried
- Covered/Smothered
- Creamed/Creamy/White Sauce/Bechamel
- Crispy/Crisped/Crunchy/Crusted
- Deluxe
- Escalloped/Scalloped
- Fricasse/Frizzled
- Fried/Deep fried
- Pesto
- Sizzled/Sizzler
- Smothered
- Stroganoff
- Stuffed
- Twice baked

Quick hint: Words ending in the letter "y" should send up red alerts, for instance: cheesy, crispy, crunchy.

Quick hint #2: If you frequent ethnic restaurants, do some research and learn those green, yellow, and red light foods, too.

10.

What's Your Favorite Non-Alcoholic Drink?

Your favorite thirst quencher might be toting a hefty dose of calories.

Water and Sports Drinks

- Gatorade: 12 ounces, 80 calories
- SoBe Lifewater: 20 ounces, 90 calories
- Glaceau Smart Water: 33.8 ounces, 0 calories
- Vitamin Water: 20 ounces, 125 calories
- Vitamin Water 10: 20 ounces, 25 calories
- Perrier (22 ounce bottle): 0 calories
- Vitamin Water Focus Kiwi-Strawberry (20 ounce bottle): 125 calories
- Hint Blackberry (16 ounce bottle): 0 calories
- Gatorade G Orange (12 ounce bottle): 80 calories
- Water (as much as you want): 0 calories

Soda and Non-Carbonated Drinks

- Mountain Dew: one 20 ounce bottle, 290 calories
- Coke Classic: one 20 ounce bottle, 233 calories
- Diet coke: one 20 ounce bottle, 0 calories
- Snapple Orangeade, 16 ounces: 200 calories
- San Pelligrino Limonata, 11.15 ounce can: 141 calories

- Can of Coke, 12 ounces: 140 calories
- Bottle of 7Up, 12 ounces: 150 calories
- Root beer float, large, 32 ounces: 640 calories

Coffee and Chocolate Drinks

- Brewed coffee, black, 16 ounce cup: 4 calories
- Home brewed coffee, cream and sugar, 16 ounces: 140 calories (average)
- Dunkin' Donuts Vanilla Bean Coolatta, 16 ounces: 430 calories
- Dunkin' Donuts Sweet Tea, 16 ounces (small): 160 calories
- Starbuck's Coffee Frappuccino, 16 ounces (grande): 240 calories
- Starbuck's Coffee Frappuccino, light, 16 ounces (grande): 110 calories
- Tazo Unsweetened Shaken Iced Passion Tea: 0 calories
- Iced Brewed Coffee with classic syrup, 12 ounces (tall): 60 calories
- Nesquick Low Fat Chocolate Milk, 8 ounce bottle: 170 calories
- Dunkin' Donuts Hot Chocolate Coolatta, 16 ounces (small): 410 calories
- Dunkin" Donuts Hot Chocolate, 14 ounces (medium regular): 320 calories
- Starbucks Mocha Frappuccino with whipped cream, 16 ounces (grande): 400 calories
- Starbucks Mocha Light Frappuccino with nonfat milk, 16 ounces (grande): 130 calories
- Iced or Hot Caffe Latte with nonfat milk, 16 ounces (grande): 90 calories
- Dunkin' Donuts Coffee Coolata made with whole milk, 16 ounces (small): 240 calories
- Dunkin' Donuts Vanilla Bean Coolatta, 16 ounces (small): 420 calories

- Dunkin' Donuts Iced Caramel Mocha Latte with milk, (large): 450 calories
- Baskin Robbins Cappuccino Blast Mocha, 16 ounces (small): 400 calories
- McDonald's McCafé Iced Caramel Mocha, 16 ounces (medium) made with whole milk and whipped cream: 300 calories
- Burger King: Iced Seattle's Best Coffee Mocha, 22 ounces (medium): 260 calories

What To Do

- Read the ingredient and nutrition labels so you know what you're getting.
- Ditch the whipped cream.
- Swap full fat or 2% milk for 1% or non-fat.
- Watch the sugar: ask for one pump instead of two, ask for sugar free syrup, add no-calorie sweetener instead of sugar, or don't sweeten at all.
- Change the size of the drink that you order: instead of a venti or an extra large, order a grande or large—or drop down to a tall, medium, or even a small-sized drink.
- Can you be satisfied with water with a hint of flavor instead of a sports drink; with iced coffee instead of a frappuccino; or with a bottle of Nesquick instead of a hot chocolate coolatta?
- If you have a two a day (or more) habit—like a hot chocolate in the morning and a frappuccino in the afternoon—substitute a plain coffee or tea (easy on the milk and sugar) or even a latte with nonfat milk for one of those choices.

11.

What To Eat When Party Food Is Heavy On Wings, Dogs, Pizza, And Chips

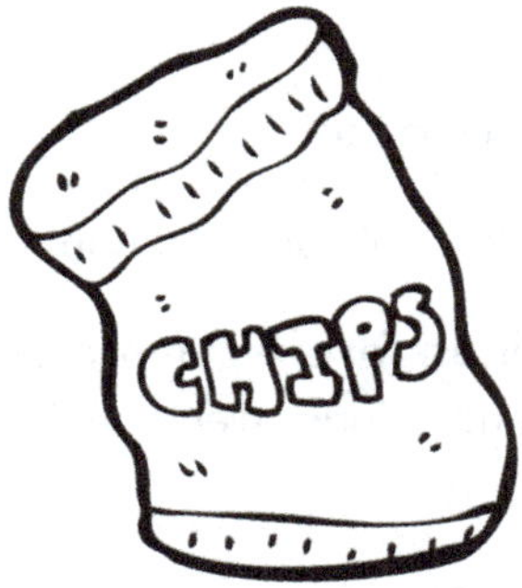

Do you look forward to the barbecue before home football games? Maybe your routine includes stopping for the fried mozzarella sticks they have every Friday night at the Student Union—or the special "American Sampler" of mozzie sticks, chicken fingers, and fried wings served on a bed of waffle fries.

Choose It And Eat It—Just Not All Of The Time

It's incredibly difficult not to eat those ooey, gooey, salty, crunchy, fatty foods when they seem to be an integral part of campus life. How many times do your senses need to be assaulted by brownies, chips, wings, cookies, or some fried delight before you give in?

Be Realistic

Saying you're never going to have (you can fill in the blank) because it's too fatty or has too many calories creates a restrictive mentality that's doomed to fail given the slimmest opportunity. Denying yourself what you love to eat—and the good times that go along with eating those special foods—probably means that it's just a matter of time until you start an eating fest that only ends when there's no more left to taste. Think of this way: what would it be like to swear that you won't eat the holiday cookies you love when you go home on break when those cookies have been a part of your holidays since you were a little kid and you baked them with your Mom?

Some guidelines for picking food at parties and tailgates:

- Stick with grilled meat, veggies, or baked chips rather than fried.
- Steer clear of salads and dressings with loads of mayonnaise—the calorie count can be huge. Look for plain or grilled veggies, or corn on the cob. If you feel you just have to have macaroni, potato, tuna, chicken, or egg salad, try to keep your portion size quite small and amp it up with tomato, onion, lettuce, and other vegetables.
- Turkey, baked ham, and grilled chicken are better choices than wings and fried chicken.
- If it isn't a tailgate without wings or barbecue, have it, enjoy it, but don't go back for seconds (certainly not for thirds).
- Plain bread, pitas, or wraps are less caloric than biscuits or cornbread.
- Go for salsa and skip the guacamole; use mustard instead of mayo.
- Minimize calories by dipping chicken wings into hot sauce instead of Buffalo sauce.

- Try using celery for crunch and as a dipper instead of chips.
- If you have pie, try to eat the filling and not the crust—that's where most of the calories are.
- Go for thin crust rather than thick crust or deep dish pizza. Choose the slices with vegetables—not pepperoni or meatballs. If you're not embarrassed, try blotting up the free-floating oil that sits on top of a greasy slice (soaking up even a teaspoon of oil saves you 40 calories and 5 grams of fat).
- Alcohol adds calories and lowers your inhibitions so your resolve not to eat everything often flies right out the window. Try alternating water or diet soda with beer or alcohol, which decreases your alcohol calories by 50%.
- You know that eventually you're going to indulge. Instead of being tempted by everything—followed by tasting everything—pick a couple of fantastic things that you love, make up your mind how much of it you're going to have (like 3 wings or 2 slices of pizza), eat it, and enjoy it.
- The key is to stick to your plan. Completely enjoy what you decide you're going to eat—but eat it and be done with it. No more triple helpings, bringing leftovers back to your room, or sneaking back into the dining hall.
- Make an informed choice. Being informed doesn't deprive you of deliciousness, but does arm you with an element of control. If you know the approximate calorie count of certain foods, you can make the best choice. For instance, perhaps you enjoy both ice cream cones and sundaes and the main thing you want is some cool creamy ice cream. If you know that a small vanilla Dairy Queen ice cream cone has 230 calories, 7g fat, 36g carbs, 6g protein and a Baskin Robbins 2 scoop hot fudge sundae is 530 calories with 29g fat, 62g carbs and 8 g of protein—which would you choose?

12.

How Much Alcohol And How Many Calories Are In Beer and Booze?

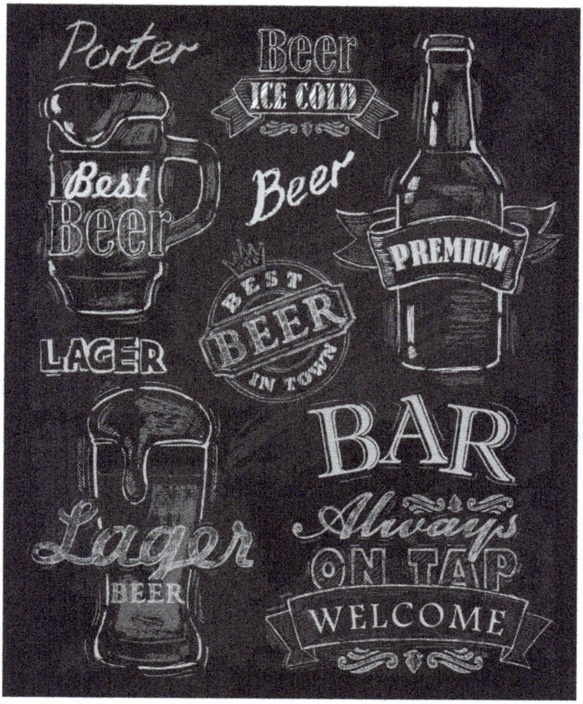

Please note: Many college students are not of legal age to purchase or drink alcoholic beverages. This book does not in any way endorse drinking alcohol by anyone under the age at which it is legally permissible to buy and consume alcoholic beverages. Facts about the amount of alcohol and calories in various types of alcoholic beverages are provided for informational purposes only.

Alcohol doesn't fill you up the way food does. Here's why: it doesn't register as "food" in your GI tract or your brain.

It doesn't fill you up, but it does have calories—7 calories a gram—more than carbs and protein which both have 4 calories a gram and fat which has 9. So, even thought it doesn't feel as though you're putting calories into your body, you can drink a lot of calories and still not feel stuffed (perhaps drunk, but not stuffed).

How Much Beer Is Equal To A Standard Drink?

A standard drink is equal to 14.0 grams (0.6 ounces) of pure alcohol, the amount usually found in:

- 12 fluid ounces of beer
- 1.5 ounces of hard liquor
- 5 ounces of wine
- 8-9 fluid ounces of malt liquor or beer with high alcohol content

Is It Safer To Have Beer Or Wine Instead Of A Drink?

No. A 12 ounce bottle of beer has about the same amount of alcohol as a 5 ounce glass of wine or a 1.5 ounce shot of liquor. Since it is the amount—not the type --of alcohol (not the amount of liquid) that you drink that affects you most, it is not safer to drink beer or wine rather than liquor.

Beer

Different types of beer and malt liquor can have very different amounts of alcohol content. Light beers can have almost as much alcohol as regular beer—about 85% as much. Put another way, on average:

- Regular beer: 5% alcohol

- Some light beers: 4.2% alcohol
- Malt liquor: 7% alcohol

<u>What's in a 12 ounce beer bottle?</u>

- Sierra Nevada Bigfoot Ale: 330 calories
- Samuel Adams Boston Lager: 180 calories
- Guinness Extra Stout: 176 calories
- Pete's Wicked Ale: 174 calories
- Harpoon IPA: 170 calories
- Heineken: 166 calories
- Killian's Irish Red: 163 calories
- Molson Ice: 160 calories
- Samuel Adams Brown Ale: 160 calories
- Budweiser: 144 calories
- Corona Light: 105 calories
- Coors Light: 102 calories
- Heineken Light: 99 calories
- Budweiser Select: 99 calories
- Miller Light: 96 calories
- Amstel Light: 95 calories
- Michelob Ultra: 95 calories
- Miller MGD 64: 64 calories
- Beck's Premier Light: 64 calories

Alcohol And Mixers

The higher the alcoholic content (proof), the greater the number of calories.

- 80-proof vodka (40% alcohol, the most common type) has 64 calories/1ounce
- 86-proof vodka (43% alcohol) has 70 calories/1 ounce

- 90-proof vodka (45% alcohol) has 73 calories/1 ounce
- 100-proof vodka (50% alcohol) has 82 calories/1 ounce

When you start adding mixers, the calories can more than double; a mixed drink runs around 250 calories.

- club soda has no calories
- 8 ounces of orange juice has 112 calories
- 8 ounces of tonic has 83 calories
- 8 ounces of ginger ale has 83 calories
- 8 ounces of tomato juice has 41 calories
- 8 ounces of classic coke has 96 calories
- 8 ounces of cranberry juice has 128 calories

Mixed drinks and fancy drinks can have a huge variation in calories.

- Frozen margarita, 12 ounces: 540 calories
- Gin and Tonic (7 ounces): 200 calories
- Mojito: (8 ounces): 214 calories
- Pina Colada (6 ounces): 378 calories
- Cosmopolitan (4 ounces): 200 calories
- Skinnygirl margarita (4 ounces): 100 calories
- Bloody Mary (5 ounces): 118 calories
- Screwdriver (8 ounces): 190 calories
- Long Island Iced Tea (8 ounces): 780 calories
- P.F. Chang China Bistro Mai Tai: 433 calories
- Rum and Coke (8 ounces): 185 calories

Calories In Wine

A standard serving of wine (5 ounces) has 125-150 calories. Many wine glasses hold much more and the amount poured into them is often significantly greater. Sweet and dessert wines have more calories than table wine and champagne.

Calories in one ounce of various wines:

- Champagne: 19 calories
- Red table wine (burgundy, cabernet): 25 calories
- Dry white wine (chablis, hock, reisling): 24 calories
- Sweet white wine (moselle, sauterne, zinfandel): 28 calories
- Rose: 20 calories
- Port (about 20% alcohol): 46 calories
- Sweet dessert wine: 47 calories
- Sangria has about 19 calories an ounce

13.

All-Nighters And 3AM Food: Some Tips

What do you eat in the middle of the night? Mostly diner food, pizza, donuts, and just about any kind of fast food: basically, cheap calories and a whole lot of fat and carbs. Slick marketing, convenience, and cheap calories really push you to order the "value meal" or to 'super-size."

There are some easy small changes you can make that won't drastically change your meal. They don't focus on skipping dessert or having a cup of broth instead of a burger, but rather on choosing to make slight alterations in what you would usually order.

Here's how to save a few calories when you eat at fast food (or fast casual) restaurants:

- Go easy on the sauce and dressings: There are lots of calories in mayo, sour cream, salad dressing and other "special" sauces, like those that come with burgers. The amount on your sandwich or salad often depends on the "hand" of the person preparing your food. The best way to control this is to ask for the sauce or dressing on the side and add it (or not) by yourself. You really can do this in fast food burger places!
- Opt for chicken or fish as long as it's not fried/breaded/or called crispy—which is just an alias for fried. Order it grilled, baked or broiled. Just be aware that lots of the sauces have a ton of sugar in them. Make your best choice (check the labels or nutrition info) and dip sparingly.

- Order your burger or chicken without bacon or cheese: A serving size of meat is 2-3 ounces—about the size of a deck of cards. You're probably getting well over that with a single meat patty. One slice of bacon adds about 43 calories, but how many sandwiches come with only one slice? One slice of American cheese clocks in at 94 calories.
- Downsize. Order a kid's meal or a junior burger. Opt for regular sizes instead of large sizes: It may seem like a good "value" but there are lots of extra calories, fat, and sugar in beefed up sizes. You'll still be satisfied. Here's a comparison. At Burger King, a Triple Whopper burger has 1,020 calories, 65g fat, 57g carbs, 3g fiber, 58g protein. You could get one of these, instead:
    - Plain regular burger: 240 calories, 8g fat, 31g carbs, 1g fiber, 12g protein (280 calories and 12g fat for a cheeseburger
    - Whopper Jr. without mayo, 1 burger: 260 calories, 10g fat, 28g carbs, 2g fiber, 13g protein
    - MorningStar Veggie Burger without mayo, 1 burger: 320 calories, 7g fat, 43g carbs, 7g fiber, 22g protein

  Do you really need (read "need" not "want") the fries, curly fries, potato sticks, or onion rings? You can order salad or a baked potato, instead (as long as you don't smother the potato in butter and/or sour cream). If you absolutely must have fries, order a small or a kid's size. Large fries can tack on around 500 calories compared to a small order at around 300 calories.
- Avoid combo specials: they might have wallet appeal but you get, on average, 55% more calories for 17% more. money. What's more important, your waistline or your wallet?
- Thin crust it: Go for a thin-crust pizza with veggies instead of a thick-crust or deep dish with meat and extra cheese.
- Skip the sides: Eating a burger or sandwich by itself is often filling enough. If you do want a side, consider ordering a fruit cup or side salad. Most fast food restaurants now offer them.

- Don't drink your calories. Soda isn't the only sugary drink. Sweetened tea, sports drinks, non-diet flavored water, juice, flavored milk, and shakes are sugary drinks, too. A 12 ounce can of coke has 140 calories and 39 grams of sugar. Eight ounces of orange juice has 110 calories and 25 grams of carbs.
- Treat yourself—but swap out your treats. Go for low-fat ice cream or frozen yogurt (be careful of the toppings), fruit popsicles, and sherbets instead of ice cream or cookies. Add sprinkles—they have a lot fewer calories than caramel or chocolate sauce.
- Salads aren't always the best pick. The dressing, the cheese, the croutons, and other mix-ins can add a ton of calories.

Don't stress too much or feel bad if your meal isn't as low in calories as you'd like. Hey, stopping for fast food is sometimes hard to avoid and it's fun to be with a crowd. Just do the best you can.

Some choices to consider:

- McDonald's Fruit 'n Yogurt Parfait, 1 parfait: 160 calories, 2g fat, 31g carbs, 4g protein
- McDonald's Apple Dippers with Low Fat Caramel Dip: 100 calories, 0.5g fat
- Subway Egg White Muffin Melts, 1 sandwich, except mega and sausage varieties): 140 - 210 calories, 3.5 - 8g fat, 18 - 20g carbs, 12 - 19g protein
- Taco Bell Fresco Chicken Soft Taco, 1 taco: 170 calories, 4g fat, 22g carbs, 12g protein
- Burger King Whopper Jr. without Mayo: 260 calories, 10g fat, 29g carbs, 13g protein
- Burger King Quaker Oatmeal, 1 order: 140 - 270 calories, 3.5 - 4g fat, 23 - 55g carbs, 3 - 5g fiber, 5g protein—the fruit topped maple flavor includes 100 calories of dried cranberries, raisins, cherries, and blueberries

- Burger King Egg & Cheese Muffin Sandwich, 1 sandwich: 220 calories, 9g fat, 22g carbs, 1g fiber, 12g protein
- KFC Grilled Chicken Breast, 1 piece: 210 calories, 8g fat, 0g carbs, 34g protein
- Carl's Jr. Hawaiian Grilled Chicken Salad, 1 salad without wontons or dressing): 260 calories, 8g fat, 34g carbs, 22g protein
- Wendy's Small Chili, 1 small order: 220 calories, 7g fat, 22g carbs, 18g protein
- Denny's Fit Fare Light Choices (under 550 calories) such as Cranberry Apple chicken Salad or Chicken Avocado Sandwich
- Dunkin" Donuts Roast Beef Pretzel Roll Sandwich: 1 sandwich: 440 calories, 7g fat

Some Choices To Think Hard About (and not in a good way):

- Taco Bell Chipotle Steak Taco Salad, 1 salad: 900 calories, 57g fat, 68g carbs, 28g protein
- Wendy's Baconator Double, 1 burger: 980 calories, 63g fat, 46g carbs, 58g protein
- Burger King Triple Whopper, 1 burger: 1,140 calories, 75g fat, 51g carbs, 67g protein
- BK Ultimate Breakfast Platter, 1 platter: 1,450 calories, 84g fat, 34g carbs, 5g fiber, 40g protein
- Denny's Macho Nacho Burger: 1020 calories, up to 1530 calories with fries
- Chili's Southwestern Chicken Pizza, 9 inches: 1550 calories
- Chicken Fajitas served with heaps of sour cream, shredded cheese, refried beans, and fried rice: (average) 1320 calories, 47 g fat.

14.

A New And Different Routine—Or Lack Of One: When Do You Eat?

Hunger is a basic survival mechanism. It's what signals your brain that your body needs nourishment and energy—and it drives you to eat for fuel. We're born with this ability—think about how babies cry when they need food—and how they stop eating when they're full.

But feeling hungry is not the only reason we eat.

Can You Train And Tame Your Hunger?

Physical—or real—hunger, the kind you feel when your stomach is growling, you're irritable as all get-out, you've got no energy and probably a throbbing headache, means your body needs food for fuel.

What To Know About Hunger

- Hunger is somewhat unpredictable. Your actual hunger levels are not the same every day and can be affected by what your body needs and does: activity, hormone levels, sickness, and other things.
- Hunger doesn't necessarily follow a time schedule. You can adjust the types and amounts of your meals to influence the next time you will be hungry. On the other hand, some people prefer to eat at the same time every day. Eating just because the hands of the clock are at noon or 6PM—even though

you're not hungry—can lead to weight gain and unhealthy eating habits.

- What you eat affects your hunger level. Carbs, fat, and protein are digested at different rates. Simple, refined carbs like soda and candy are digested rapidly. They give you quick energy from a surge in your blood sugar—which is followed by a rapid drop in your energy. Protein foods give you the most sustained blood sugar levels and satiety without the blood sugar spikes.
- Eating food that has a balance of protein, carbs, and healthy fats is probably the best way to give your body the fuel it needs, to satisfy your hunger, and to keep you feeling full longer.
- The amount you eat at a meal affects you hunger levels since larger meals take longer to digest. Haven't you ever eaten so much for dinner that you're not hungry until lunch the next day?
- When you eat small meals you'll get hungry more often and perhaps fuel your body more efficiently—which is why some people prefer 5 or 6 small meals a day rather than two or three larger ones.

All kinds of foods can play a role in satisfying your hunger. Labeling food good or bad puts the food in charge. Depriving yourself of a particular food or attaching special meaning to it can set you up for cravings and overeating. Allow yourself to make good choices from all foods, to eat when you're hungry, and to eat portions that satisfy but don't stuff you. This puts you, not the food, in charge.

15.

What Real Hunger Feels Like: How To Tell If You're Really Hungry Enough To Eat

Real hunger produces true physical feelings –not just a desire to eat. This is what real hunger feels like in your body:

- You feel like you have to eat right away
- You're having trouble concentrating
- You're irritable
- You're low on energy or really tired
- You have a headache
- You might be nauseated
- Your stomach is growling or you have a gnawing feeling

There are a number of biochemical and physical factors that are responsible for true hunger. The two primary ones come from your blood sugar and your stomach.

Your stomach, about the size of your fist, is a muscle that can expand and contract. When it contracts (because it's empty) you may have a growling empty feeling, hunger pangs, or maybe nausea.

Glucose, also called blood sugar, is what your body uses for energy. Your brain relies primarily on glucose for fuel to function. Your hunger symptoms are directly affected by whether or not there's a sufficient level of blood glucose available for fuel.

With low blood sugar you feel like you have no energy, you can't concentrate, you're irritable, you may have a headache, and you can be lightheaded. Other things can cause these feelings, too, so it's important to make sure that they're coming from low blood sugar. A way to do that is to figure out if they go away when you eat.

There's Head Hunger, Too!

Head hunger, or psychological hunger, usually doesn't have physical symptoms and can happen at any time. It often provokes emotional eating—usually in response to gremlins like stress, sadness, loneliness, anger, fear, or boredom.

Head hunger (eatouteatwell.com/head hunger) also serves as a distraction—the eating it provokes can be a way to distract you from difficult situations, projects, and encounters. It's triggered by habits like watching TV, working on the computer or driving in the car, food cravings, or as a need to procrastinate. Whatever triggers your head hunger can make you think you're hungry when you're really not.

Sometimes we become disconnected from the signals that let us know when we're hungry or when we're full and satisfied. Some of us don't even feel hungry because we eat so frequently that we never get to the point when we feel real hunger. Remember that true, real hunger is a physical sensation, not a thought.

The Hunger Scale

There's a hunger scale that can help you identify how hungry you are before, during, and after eating. The scale goes from 1 to 10. At 1 you're ravenous and at 10 you're so full that you feel sick.

The Scale:

1. You're ravenous and too hungry to give a hoot about what you eat

2. You're starving and absolutely must eat immediately because you're irritable, cranky, and have no energy
3. You're hungry and the urge to eat is strong
4. Your hunger pangs are signaling the first signs of hunger; you're a little hungry
5. You're satisfied—not hungry but not full—and you're not aware of food sitting in your stomach
6. You're fully satisfied and are aware of food sitting in your stomach
7. You're very full, your stomach feels stretched, you're past the point of satisfaction but can still find room for more
8. You're uncomfortable because your stomach is too full and you really wish you hadn't had those last few bites
9. You're stuffed, very uncomfortable, and your clothes feel very tight—the snap on your jeans doesn't stand a chance
10. You're beyond full and feel sick, miserable, and you don't want to move

What Number?

- If you're at number 5 or above you're probably not physically hungry and something else is triggering your eating.
- If you're at number 4 you can wait to eat or eat a little bit.
- If you're at 2 or 3 it's a good time to eat—have you noticed that food tastes pretty good when you're hungry?
- If you're at number 1 you need to eat—but pay attention to what you're doing. When you're starving you don't care too much about what or how much you eat—and usually shovel food in as quickly as possible—which can result in overeating (pigging out) and landing at a 7 and up.
- Gauge your hunger. If you're only a little hungry, only eat a little. Preventive eating—or eating because you might be hungry in a little while—can pack in a lot of calories.

16.

Concession Stands And Stadium Food: Good, Better, And Best Choices

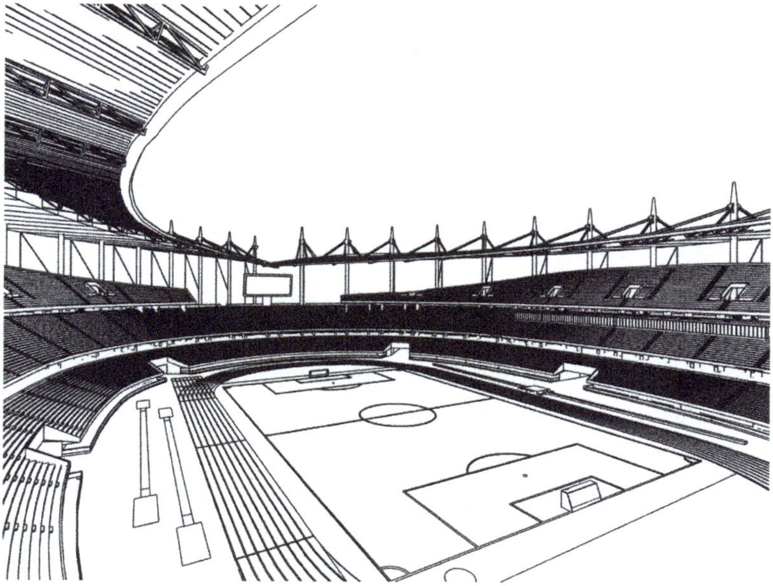

Oh, the choices! How can you possibly not chow down on thousands of calories when there are food vendors or tailgating friends about every 20 feet hawking dogs, barbecue, burgers, and fried everything?

There Are Ways And Then There Are Ways

If you've got a will of iron you could ignore the food and drinks. But if you're tempted at every turn, try to minimize the damage without taking away the fun. If you know you're going to be having a stadium or concession stand meal, do some thinking, planning, and sleuthing. The best choices are not always the obvious ones. If you always eat sausage and peppers at the stadium or corn dogs from your favorite concession stand, plan for it, have it, and enjoy it.

But give the total picture some thought. Do you need both peanuts and popcorn? Can you make do with a regular hot dog instead of a foot-long? Can you choose the small popcorn instead of the jumbo tub? Can you ditch the soda—or maybe the second one—and replace it with water?

Make Your Best Choice

Use these facts as guidelines:

- Cotton Candy: Nothing but heated and colored sugar that's spun into threads with added air. Cotton candy on a stick or wrapped around a paper cone (about an ounce) has around 105 calories; a 2 ounce bag (common size) has 210. A lot of sugar, but not a lot of calories—albeit empty ones.

- Funnel cake: The fried dough wonder is made by pouring dough through a funnel into cooking oil and deep frying the "funnels" of dough until they're golden-brown and crispy—then topping the pieces with powdered sugar, syrup, or honey. The calories vary enormously depending on the quantity and toppings. Regardless of the shape, they're all dough fried in oil topped with a sweetener—which means high calories and low nutrition. You have to figure a minimum of around 300 calories for a 6 inch funnel cake (do they ever come that small?).

- Cracker Jack (officially cracker jack, not jacks): candy-coated popcorn with some peanuts. A 3.5 ounce stadium size box has 420 calories but it does have 7g of protein and 3.5g of fiber.

- Hamburger: 6 ounces of food stand beef (they're not using extra lean—the more fat, the juicier it is) on a bun has about 490 calories—without cheese or other toppings—which up the ante.

- Grilled Chicken Sandwich: 6 ounces, 280 calories—not a bad choice. 6 ounces of chicken tenders clock in at 446 calories. Barbecue dipping sauce adds 30 calories a tablespoon.
- Hot Dog: A regular hot dog with mustard has about 290 calories—that's 180 for the 2 ounce dog, 110 for the bun, zilch for regular yellow mustard. Two tablespoons of sauerkraut adds another 5-10 calories and a punch of flavor, 2 tablespoons of ketchup adds 30, and 2 tablespoons of relish another 40. A Nathan's hot dog racks up 320 calories; a foot-long Hebrew National 510 calories. A regular size corn dog has around 280 calories.
- Fried Battered Clams: One cup (5 large clams or 8 medium clams or 10 small clams) has around 222 calories.
- Pizza: Stadium pizza is usually larger than a regular slice, about 1/6 of a 16-inch pie (instead of 1/8) making it about 435 calories a slice—add calories if you add toppings.
- Super Nachos with Cheese: A 12 ounce serving (40 chips, 4 ounces of cheese) has about 1,500 calories!!! Plain French fries look like a caloric bargain by comparison.
- French Fries: A large serving has about 500 calories. A serving of Hardee's chili cheese fries has 700 calories and 350 of them come from fat.
- Potato Chips: One single serving bag has 153 calories (94 of them from fat).
- Peanuts in the Shell: An 8 ounce bag has 840 calories; a 12 ounce bag has 1,260. Yes, they have some protein and fiber. But wow on the calories.
- Soft Pretzel: One large soft pretzel has 483 calories—giant soft pretzels (7-8 ounces) have about 700 calories.
- Draft Beer: A stadium draft beer—a 20 ounce cup, the usual size—has about 240 calories. A light draft saves you 60 calories.
- Coca Cola: A 12 ounce can has 140 calories and close to 10 teaspoons of sugar.

- Good Humor Ice Cream: Strawberry Shortcake Ice Cream Bar (83g): 230 calories; Toasted Almond (113g): 240 calories; Candy Center Crunch: 310 calories; Low Fat Ice Cream Sandwich, vanilla:130 calories
- Helmet Ice Cream: Your team's mini-helmet filled with swirly Carvel, 550-590 calories.
- Popcorn: FYI—at Yankee Stadium a jumbo size has 1,484 calories and a souvenir bucket has 2,473 calories.

17.

Can You Save Calories Eating A Ham And Cheese Sandwich Instead Of A Salad?

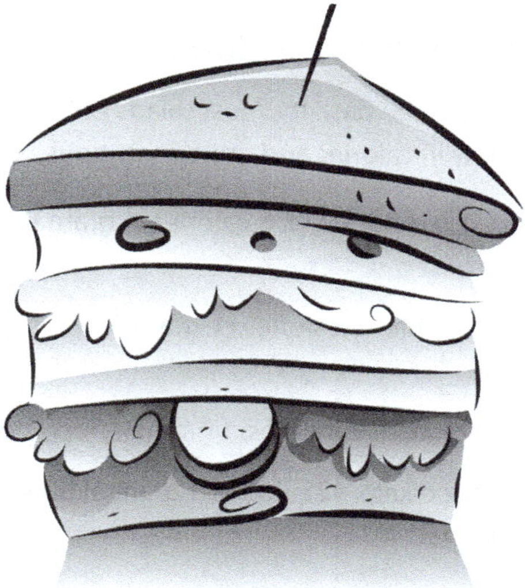

A ham and cheese sandwich (or turkey or roast beef) is always a good default when you're stuck. But do you think twice about ordering a sandwich instead of a salad?

So many of us think a salad, instead of a sandwich, is the way to go if we're trying to be calorie conscious. Somehow we've embraced the idea that salads are always a light and healthy choice. Sometimes they are—but all too often they aren't.

Sometimes a sandwich is the clear winner in terms of calories and fat. A ham and cheese sandwich ranges from 350 to 450 calories depending upon how much ham and cheese there really is, the type of bread, and whether it comes with mustard or mayo (and, of course, without fries or chips).

And sometimes the salad is a better choice—depending on what goes into it. The nutrient rich plant foods that make the base of a salad are high in antioxidants—especially the dark green, orange, and red vegetables. Most of the vegetables are full of fiber—good for your health and for keeping you feel fuller for a longer period of time. And salads take a long time to eat—much longer than sandwiches or pizza that you can scarf down far more quickly.

The Green Base For Salads

The green stuff that's the base for most salads isn't the problem. Most greens are very low in calories and pretty nutritious.

- 1 cup shredded Romaine: 8 calories, 1 gram fiber, 1 gram protein, 0 gram fat
- 1 cup of Arugula: 6 calories, 1 gram fiber, 1 gram protein, 0 gram fat
- 1 cup raw spinach: 7 calories, 1 gram of fiber, 1 gram protein
- 1 cup chopped kale: 32 calories, 1 gram of fiber, 2 grams of protein, 0 gram fat

Salad Add-Ins:

High calorie add-ins and dressings can make salads a "no thank you" choice instead of a filling, healthy choice. Choose wisely—but don't eliminate taste, flavor, and protein for the sake of calories. You'll just end up unsatisfied—and hungry!

- Most salad dressing ladles hold three to four tablespoons and many people have been known to use two ladles worth of dressing on their salads. Creamy dressing has 72 calories in a tablespoon, ranch has 73, Caesar has 78, and generic "salad dressing has 60. That's in a tablespoon—you could be pouring 8 tablespoons of dressing on your salad. You do the math.

- Tuna, macaroni, egg, and chicken salads, the holy grail of delis and salad bars, are loaded with mayonnaise. On average (for a half cup): chicken salad has around 208 calories, 16g of fat; tuna salad has 192 calories, 9g fat; tuna pasta salad has 250 calories, 9g fat; macaroni salad has 170 calories, 9g fat. (Remember, ½ cup is pretty small.)
- Then there's cheese. A ¼ cup (which is really small) serving of shredded cheddar has 114 calories, 9g fat; blue cheese has 80 calories, 6g fat; feta has 75 calories, 6g fat.
- Croutons and Crispy Noodles: ¼ cup of plain croutons has 31 calories, 0g fat; 1 serving of McDonald's Butter Garlic Croutons has 60 calories, 1g fat; ¼ cup of crispy noodles has 74 calories, 4g fat
- Dried cranberries: ¼ cup has 98 calories, 0g fat
- Nuts and seeds: ¼ cup sunflower seeds: 210 calories, 19g fat; chopped walnuts: 193 calories, 18g fat
- Avocado, ¼ cup: 58 calories, 5g fat
- Bacon bits, 1 tablespoon: 25 calories, 2g fat
- Bread (often used to sop up leftover dressing): 1 piece of French bread has 82 calories, 1g fat; 1 dinner roll, 78 calories, 2g fat. Dressing sopped up by the bread or roll: lots of extra fat calories!

18.

Seven Ways To Cut Down On Pizza Calories

"Let's order pizza." Familiar words? Take comfort that you fit the stats: American men, women, and children eat, on average, 46 slices (eatouteatwell.com/slices of pizza) of pizza a year.

The Good And The Not-So-Good

It's difficult to estimate the number of calories and fat grams in a slice of pizza because the size, the type of crust, and the amount of cheese, meat, or other toppings vary enormously.

Here's the good news: pizza can be a healthy food choice filled with complex carbs, B-vitamins, calcium, protein, vitamin A, and vitamin C and calorically okay if you choose wisely and don't eat more than your fair share.

The not so good news: the amount of fat, calories, and portion size. If your mouth starts to water at the thought of golden brown crust and cheesy goodness remember that a slice of pizza should be about the size of two dollar bills—not the size of a small frying pan or a quarter of a 12" circle.

7 Ways To Build a Better Slice of Pizza

1. Order thin crust rather than a thick crust or deep dish.
2. Resist the urge to ask for double cheese—better yet, go light on the cheese or use reduced-fat cheese (if they have it).

3. Ask for a pizza without cheese but topped with veggies and a little olive oil. You can always sprinkle on a little grated parmesan for flavor; one tablespoon has only 22 calories.
4. Instead of cheese go for big flavors like onion, garlic, olives but use them somewhat sparingly because of the oil. And don't forget anchovies—a lot of flavor for minimal calories—but you have to like them!
5. Choose vegetable toppings instead of meat (think about the fat content in sausage, pepperoni, and meatballs) and you might shave 100 calories from your meal. Pile on veggies like mushrooms, peppers, olives, tomatoes, onion, broccoli, spinach, and asparagus. Some places have salad pizza—great if it's not loaded with oil.
6. Order a side salad (careful with the dressing) and cut down on the amount of pizza. Salad takes longer to eat, too.
7. If you're willing (and not embarrassed or grossed out), try blotting up the free-floating oil that sits on top of a greasy slice with a napkin. Blotting (it's easy to do this on the kind of hot slice where the oil runs down your arm when you pick it up) can soak up a teaspoon of oil worth 40 calories and 5 grams of fat.

So You Know:

Domino's: compare the calories in the same size pizza but with different types of crusts and fillings:

14 inch large classic hand-tossed pizza:

- America's Favorite (Peperoni, mushroom, sausage, 1/8 of pizza): 390 calories
- Bacon Cheeseburger (Beef, bacon, cheddar cheese), 1/8 of pizza: 420 calories
- Vegi Feast (Green pepper, onion, mushroom, black olive, extra cheese, 1/8 of pizza): 340 calories

14 inch large ultimate deep dish pizza:

- America's Favorite (Peperoni, mushroom, sausage), 1/8 of pizza: 400 calories
- Bacon Cheeseburger (Beef, bacon, cheddar cheese), 1/8 of pizza: 430 calories
- Vegi Feast (Green pepper, onion, mushroom, black olive, extra cheese), 1/8 of pizza: 350 calories

14 inch large crunchy thin crust pizza:

- America's Favorite (Peperoni, mushroom, sausage, 1/8 of pizza: 280 calories)
- Bacon Cheeseburger (Beef, bacon, cheddar cheese), 1/8 of pizza: 310 calories
- Vegi Feast (Green pepper, onion, mushroom, black olive, extra cheese), 1/8 of pizza: 230 calories

Domino add-ons:

- Breadstick, 1 stick, no sauce, 130 calories
- Cheesy Bread, 1 stick, no sauce: 140 calories
- Cinna Stix, 1 stick, no sauce, 140 calories
- Marinara Dipping Sauce, container for 8 sticks, 25 calories
- Garlic Dipping Sauce, container for 8 sticks: 440 calories
- Sweet Icing Dipping Sauce, container for 8 sticks: 250 calories

Mall Pizza Can Be Okay—And Not Okay

Per slice:

- Sbarro's Low Carb Cheese Pizza: 310 calories, 14g fat
- Sbarro's Low Carb Sausage/Pepperoni Pizza: 560 calories, 35g fat
- Sbarro's Fresh Tomato Pizza: 450 calories, 14g fat
- Sbarro's "Gourmet" pizzas: between 610 and 780 calories, more than 20g fat
- Costco Food Court Pepperoni Pizza: 620 calories, 30g fat
- "Stuffed" pizzas: 790 calories minimum, over 33g fat

19.

Snacks Are Good But Are You Eating A Snack Or Another Meal?

We chow down on a lot of snack food everyday—25% of our calories—that's a quarter of our food—come from them! During long paper writing spells or study sessions snacking can be a 24/7 activity—and can make up a very significant portion of your daily food.

Thoughtful, planned snacking:

- can keep you from feeling outrageously hungry, really grouchy, and needing to take a midday nap
- can put the brakes on hitting every food stand in the dining hall
- will help keep your metabolism revved up—there's a school of thought that believes you burn more calories over the course of a day if you eat a small meal or snack every 3 to 4 hours

What's A Snack?

An individual snack isn't a fourth meal (eatouteatwell.com/fourth meal). It should be between 150 and 200 calories, have at least 8 grams of protein and 3 grams of fiber to fill you up and help maintain a stable blood sugar. Keep the fat and sugar grams low.

Beware health halo foods—the so-called "healthy" snacks that are really a bunch of sugar and/or fat in disguise. Examples are certain (but not all) types of cereals, breakfast and protein bars, yogurt-covered anything (like raisins and pretzels), sports and energy drinks, smoothies, and frozen yogurt. Check labels, you might be surprised.

If you're not hungry, don't snack. Ask yourself if you're snacking because of hunger, habit, or some other reason—like boredom or too much family togetherness.

Some Snack Ideas:

Pick snacks that taste good and you look forward to eating. Some good choices:

- Baby carrots (or other vegetables) and hummus.
- Half a cup of cottage cheese with fruit or whole grain crackers.
- An apple, orange, pear, peach, or grapes or berries with ¼ cup of almonds or reduced-fat cheese or a low-fat cheese stick.
- Whole-grain crackers, a slice of whole grain bread, or a banana with peanut butter.
- A combination of nuts, seeds, raisins, and whole grain cereal (without the M&Ms). Be careful of portions—although they're healthy, nuts are a higher calorie food.
- A whole wheat or multi-grain English muffin with a small amount of nut or seed butter.
- Low-fat or non-fat yogurt with raisins, a banana, or a small amount of whole grain cereal.
- A 12 ounce skim latte or cappuccino, hot or iced.
- Various nut or protein bars—check the ingredients and nutrition labels.
- Various kinds of jerky, which is high in protein and quite lean. A deterrent might be the preservatives in some brands.

20.

Are You Eating Sugar When You Think You Aren't: Carbs Are Both Simple And Complex

Carbohydrates, carbs for short, are the sugars, starches, and fiber we eat. Except for fiber, carbs get transformed by your body into blood sugar, mostly glucose, your body's basic fuel.

"Carbs" usually conjure up images of sugary candy or baked goods, but an enormous number of foods—lots of them healthy—contain carbs. They're the main energy source for your body and the main source of calories in just about every culture's diet. Carbs and protein have four calories per gram; fat has nine calories per gram and alcohol has seven.

Does The Type Of Carb Matter?

Which of these foods contain lots of carbs: fruit juice, table sugar, non-fat milk, bananas, blueberries, hamburger buns, multi-grain bread, pumpkin pie, popcorn, scones, corn, Hershey's kisses, honey, sweet potatoes? If you chose them all, bingo!

The calories per gram in carbs are the same whether they come from chocolate or oranges. Since most carbs are broken down into glucose does it really matter which kind you eat? Or, said another way, is the energy (calories) in a teaspoonful of sugar any better or worse than the energy in peas, potatoes, or Pepsi?

If You're Looking For A Simple Answer—It's Complex

Most carbs come from plant-based foods: fruit, veggies, grains, and legumes (lentils, peas, beans, peanuts). The only animal based foods with lots of carbs are dairy products.

Simple carbs are sugars like the glucose and fructose in fruit and some veggies; the lactose in milk; and the sucrose from cane or beet sugar.

Refined carbs or simple sugars—like those found in candy and baked and processed goods made with refined white flour—are digested rapidly and often cause your blood sugar to elevate quickly and then drop leaving you feeling tired, irritable, and craving more sugar to get your blood sugar levels back up again. Sugars added to many processed foods account for a large portion of the simple carbs we eat and are a big reason that sugar makes up 16% of all calories Americans consume (it was 11% twenty years ago).

Complex carbs are chains of simple sugars. They're primarily the starches and the fiber found in plant foods like grains and grain products (bread, pasta), beans, potatoes, and corn.

Which Is Preferable?

The answer isn't totally straightforward. A lot of foods high in sugar, especially the ones with added sugars, qualify as "empty calories," foods with lots of calories and few nutrients.

Complex carbs usually come with a suitcase filled with nutritional extras. Try to choose the complex carb version of a food, for instance the whole fruit with fiber is better than just the juice. Whole grains (think brown rice instead of white, multi-grain bread instead of white sandwich buns or rolls) are more nutritious than refined grains because they still have the bran and the germ, parts often removed in refined grains. Because of this they are digested more slowly and have a more gentle effect on your blood sugar.

Because of their fiber content, the same is true for vegetables and beans. Dairy products and fruit both contain simple carbs, but because of the other nutrients they contain, they're also an important part of a healthy diet.

What's Added Sugar?

Natural sugars are found in foods like milk and yogurt (lactose), in fruit (fructose), and many other foods.

Added sugar doesn't occur naturally but is added during food processing, preparation, or at the table. Nutrition labels don't differentiate between natural and added sugars. You have to look for sugar in the food's ingredient list. Added sugars have no nutritional value other than calories.

Americans average 475 calories (eatouteatwell.com/added sugars) from added sugars every day, a lot more than the recommended daily max of 100 calories (6 teaspoons) from added sugars for women and 150 calories (9 teaspoons) for men. Think of it this way, that extra 475 calories of sugar is the equivalent of 30 teaspoons of sugar a day.

The Sugar Masquerade

Sugar masquerades under many different names and in many forms. You know that candy, cookies, and soda have sugar in them and you know when you're dousing your pancakes with syrup or dumping packages of sugar into your coffee. But, who thinks of hamburger buns and crackers—or even ice cream or canned fruit—in terms of teaspoons of sugar? (Check the ingredients!)

Some other names for sugar (there are more, too):

- Dextrose, glucose, fructose, lactose, maltose (typical sugars end in –ose)
- Brown, raw, or invert sugar and/or "syrup"

- Honey
- Corn syrup, high fructose corn syrup
- Maltodextrin
- Fruit juice concentrate
- Molasses
- Invert sugar
- Sorghum
- Agave nectar
- Maple syrup, malt syrup, brown rice syrup
- Cane sugar, evaporated cane juice

Sweet Labels (eatouteatwell.com/sweet labels):

- **Sugar free** means there is less than 0.5 grams of sugar per serving
- **No sugar added** means sugar or ingredients that substitute for sugar, like fruit juices or honey, can't be added during packaging or processing. But ingredients used in the recipe, like chocolate chips, might be the full sugar kind.

21.

Are You Being Duped By Labels: Is Reduced Fat Really Low Fat?

Are labels that scream "low in fat" or "fat-free" pulling the wool over your eyes? Packaged food labels list the ingredients in a product in descending order by weight, not quantity. The first ingredient listed has the greatest amount by weight; the last ingredient is the one with the least amount by weight. That's why preservatives are usually at the end of the ingredients list; a ton of chemicals aren't necessary to increase shelf life—a little bit will do it. Fat, sugar, and grains have more heft so they're usually closer to the beginning of the ingredients list.

A Primer On Nutrition Labels: Fatty To Lean

Fatty Labels

Labels have to include the total amount of fat, saturated fat and unsaturated fat, which paves the way for the low, reduced, and fat free categories.

- **Low fat** means 3 grams of fat or less per serving (or per 100 grams of food)
- **Reduced fat** means the food product contains 50% (or less) of the fat found in the regular version
- **Less fat** means 25% or less fat than the comparison food
- **Fat free** means the product has less than 0.5 grams of fat per serving, with no added fat or oil

The Low Down On Low, Light (Lite), Lean, And Reduced Calories

- **Reduced calorie on the label** means at least 25% fewer calories per serving than in the regular (full calorie) version of the product
- **Low calorie** means there are 40 calories or less per serving and less than 0.4 calories per gram of food
- **Light (fat)** means 50% or less of the fat than in the regular, full calorie, version
- **Light (calories)** means 1/3 fewer calories than the regular, full calorie version
- **Lean** (meat, poultry or seafood) means less than 10 grams of fat, 4.5 grams of saturated fat, and 95 mg of cholesterol in a 100 gram serving
- **Extra lean** (meat, poultry or seafood) means less than 5 grams of fat, 2 grams of saturated fat, and 95 mg of cholesterol in a 100 gram serving

What To Do

A product sporting a reduced fat label means that it contains at least 25% less fat than the original version, which doesn't necessarily mean that it ends up being a low-fat product.

Take a reduced fat muffin. If the fat content in the original full fat muffin is 30g but in the reduced fat version the fat has been reduced to 15g, that's a 50% reduction which allows it to say it is a reduced fat product. But, that reduced fat muffin still has a fat content five times higher than the 3g of fat per serving that officially qualifies it as low fat.

Here's another kicker: According to the FDA, a food can be labeled fat free if it contains less than 0.5 grams of fat per serving. So, something could have 0.49 grams of fat and still be called fat free.

Maybe you're saying, "so what." Here's the issue: you're probably eating more than one serving—a serving is often smaller than what most of us eat. If a serving has 0.4 grams of fat, it can be labeled "fat free"—but, if you're eating 3 servings (not such a stretch of the imagination), you're actually eating 1.2 grams of fat (3 x 0.4 grams) in a food that's labeled "fat free." 1.2 grams of fat isn't a huge amount—but it illustrates that it's good to read and understand what labels mean so you know what you're getting in your food.

22. Ice Cream And Frozen Yogurt: How Big Are The Bowls?

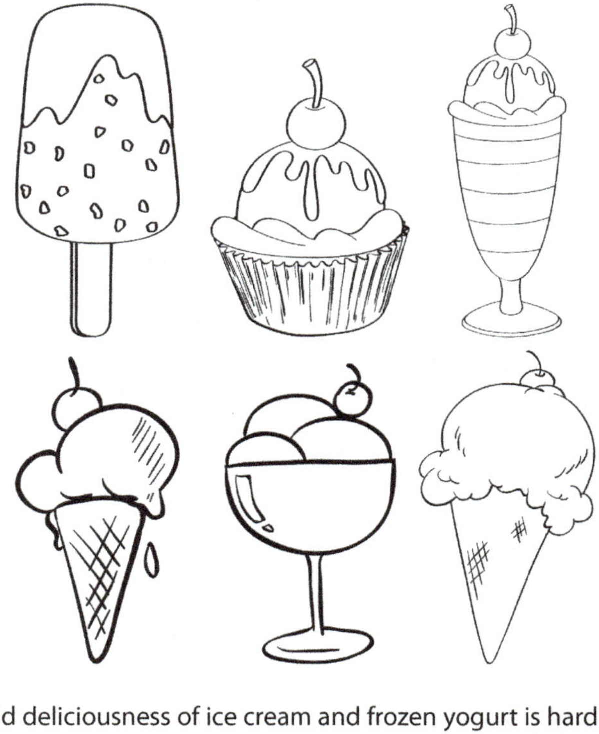

The cold deliciousness of ice cream and frozen yogurt is hard to beat. There are an astounding number of choices with varying amounts of fat, sugar, and calories. The sad truth is that no matter how innovative food scientists and savvy marketers have become, a three-scoop sundae with hot fudge, whipped cream, and other assorted toppings still isn't going to rank at the top of the health-o-meter.

Ice Cream Vs. Gelato

Ice cream means different things in different countries. In the US the government regulates what can be called ice cream, but in some other countries ice cream can mean all frozen desserts.

Ice cream and its relative, gelato (eatouteatwell.com/ice cream and gelato), are usually dairy-based. The main differences are in texture, fat and air content, and ingredients. Gelato, made and stored at a higher temperature than ice cream, is softer, smoother, and quicker to melt. Both are usually made from sugar, milk, eggs, and flavorings.

Gelato has a higher sugar content and less butterfat than ice cream, usually about 4 to 8% compared to ice cream's 10 to 20%. The sugar/water combination acts like anti-freeze and prevents the gelato from freezing solid.

Both ice cream and gelato are churned during the freezing process, which incorporates air. Most commercial ice cream contains about 50% air while gelato contains much less, generally 20-35%.

Frozen Yogurt

Milk and milk by-products are the main ingredients in frozen yogurt.

Frozen yogurt companies have their own recipes, but most common frozen yogurts contain yogurt cultures, sweetener, corn syrup, milk solids, gelatin, flavoring, and coloring.

Sugar makes up 15-17% of frozen yogurt and adds flavor, body, and thickness. Because it's made with milk instead of cream, frozen yogurt is lower in fat than most ice creams. Most of the nonfat "original" or "plain" flavors are usually the lowest in calories at about 30-35 calories per ounce with about 20g of sugar.

Frozen yogurt wears a healthy food "halo" but doesn't always warrant one. Some varieties are "healthier" than others—depending on the company's recipe and the quality and quantity of ingredients and added toppings.

Frozen Desserts (eatouteatwell.com/frozen desserts):

- Federal standards say that to be called ice cream (eatouteatwell.com/ice cream) a frozen dessert must have a minimum of 10% milk fat. Economy brands usually have the least and super premium brands have more. Less than 10% makes it ice milk or light ice cream. Frozen yogurt, which isn't regulated by the FDA, but is by some states, might or might not contain live bacterial cultures.
- Premium ice cream has between 11% and 15% butterfat, which makes it richer, denser, higher in calories. It often comes in gourmet flavors.
- Regular ice cream—what you usually find in the larger containers in the market—is somewhat less dense and contains 10% to 11% butterfat (perfect for milkshakes).
- Economy ice cream, by law, has 10% butterfat.
- Light ice cream has either 50% less fat or 33% fewer calories than the producer's regular ice cream. Here's the hitch: because it starts with fat content, light versions of premium ice cream can have more fat and calories than the regular version of other brands.
- Reduced fat ice cream must, by law, have 25% less fat than the regular ice cream produced by the same vendor.
- Soft serve ice cream is the same as regular ice cream but is served at a higher temperature.
- French Style Ice Cream also called glace, has a custard base that includes eggs, which makes it silky and rich.
- Gelato (plural, gelati) has more milk than cream (if any) so its fat content is significantly lower. It doesn't saturate your taste buds as much as ice cream so the flavor seems more intense. Gelato, served at a higher temperature than ice cream, usually looks more like frozen yogurt or whipped cream than ice cream.

How Many Calories?

Here are the general caloric ranges for "naked" ice cream, gelato, and frozen yogurt (without sauce, toppings, nuts, and whipped cream).

- 3.5 ounces of milk-based gelato has between 120 and 160 calories, 4g to 8g fat, 30g to 45g of carbs, 3g to 5g protein
- 3.5 ounces of American ice cream (not churned, light, or reduced fat) averages 240 calories, 15g fat, and 24g carbs
- 3.5 ounces of light ice cream can vary between 100 to close to 200 calories depending upon whether it's just light or slow churned light

Frozen Yogurt

- Despite different recipes, frozen yogurts are fairly comparable in calories. One-half cup of Pinkberry has 116 calories, 0g fat and 20g of sugar; TCBY's 98% fat free vanilla has 120 calories, 2g fat, and 17g of sugar; Ben & Jerry's vanilla frozen yogurt has 130 calories, 1.5g fat, and 16g of sugar.
- One cup of low-fat frozen yogurt runs about 210 calories. More specifically, for a one cup serving:
    - Frozen yogurt: Calories: 214; Fat: 2.94g; Carbs: 39.24g; Protein: 9.40g
    - Nonfat frozen yogurt: Calories: 164; Fat: 0.65g; Carbs: 34.84g; Protein: 5.96g
    - Low fat frozen yogurt: 214 calories, 2.94g fat, 39.24g carbs, 9.40g protein
    - Chocolate frozen yogurt (soft serve): 230 calories, 8.64g fat, 35.86g carbs, 5.76g protein
    - Vanilla frozen yogurt (soft serve): 234 calories, 8.06g fat, 34.84g carbs, 5.76g protein
    - Frozen yogurt (non-chocolate flavors): 210 calories, 2.70g fat, 38.24g carbs, 9.14g protein

- Chocolate frozen yogurt (not soft serve): 226 calories; 3.90g fat; 43.22g carbs, 10.48g protein
- Frozen flavored yogurt (non-chocolate, not self serve): 221 calories, 6.26g fat, 37.58g carbs, 5.22g protein
- Nonfat chocolate frozen yogurt: Calories: 172 calories, 1.32g fat, 35.19g carbs, 8.95g protein

What To Do

- Get a small serving of ice cream. Even if you indulge in your favorite full-fat flavor, you'll save as many as 550 calories with a 5-ounce size instead of a 12-ounce. Ditto with cones. One scoop has a lot fewer calories than two or three. You get the same taste and flavor and will most likely be completely satisfied. When you start with a smaller cup rather than a large one, you're already ahead of the game. Despite the fact that you swear you won't fill up a large cup, you almost always do.

- Reverse the order of what you put into your cup. Put the ice cream, gelato or yogurt on top, not under, the layered toppings. Make space-filling low calorie fruit like berries or fresh pineapple your first layer. Then add things with crunch and volume, like cereal. Follow with the frozen stuff, then perhaps a sprinkling of candy crunch on top. Starting with yogurt or ice cream often means putting a lot of it in the cup followed by a lot of toppings. Putting lower calorie food with a lot of volume on the bottom takes up space and can save calories.

- Try not to mix flavors. Swirling a couple is fun, but taste buds are funny. When you pick just one flavor your taste buds are happy and you probably end up feeling more satisfied than if you have a variety of flavors.

23.

Some Lower Calorie Alternatives If You Like Frozen Desserts With Toppings Instead Of Naked

You can put just about anything on ice cream, gelato, and frozen yogurt and someone, somewhere in the world, has probably chosen some pretty random and unique toppings to put on their plain old vanilla.

Toppings Can Add A Mountain Of Calories

The problem is that the standard fare—toppings like hot fudge, whipped cream, peanuts, walnuts in syrup, crushed heath bar, caramel sauce—can add hundreds of calories and not much nutrition.

Stats for some common ice cream toppings:

- Smucker's Spoonable Hot Fudge Topping: 2 tablespoons, 140 calories
- Smucker's Spoonable Ice Cream Topping Pecans in Syrup Topping: 1 tablespoon, 170 calories
- Regular Redi Whip: 2 tablespoons, 20 calories
- Cool Whip, extra creamy: 2 tablespoons, 32 calories

- Regular M&M's: 10 pieces,103 calories
- Peanut M&M's: about 16 pieces, 200 calories

Some Standbys That Are Lower In Calories

- Rainbow Sprinkles (Mr. Sprinkles): 1 teaspoon, 20 calories
- Chocolate Sprinkles (jimmies): 1 tablespoon, 35 calories
- Smucker's Spoonable Ice Cream Topping, Light Hot Fudge, Fat Free: 2 tablespoons, 90 calories
- 10 mini marshmallows: 22 calories

Think Outside The Box For Lower Calorie Choices

Why not think about fruit, cereal, or a crushed up 100-calorie pack of anything? Here are some other suggestions:

- Smucker's Spoonable Pineapple Topping: 2 tablespoons, 100 calories
- Fat Free Redi Whip: 2 tablespoons, 5 calories
- Cool whip, light: 2 tablespoons, 16 calories
- Cool Whip, fat-free: 2 tablespoons, 15 calories
- 1 mini box of raisins (.5 ounces): 42 calories
- One medium banana: 105 calories
- One cup strawberry halves: 49 calories
- Sugar-free Jello pudding: 60 calories

<u>Fruit (fresh and not), once ounce serving:</u>

- Strawberries: 9 calories
- Blueberries: 16 calories
- Blackberries: 12 calories
- Rasberries: 15 calories
- Pineapple: 17 calories

- Mango: 17 calories
- Grated sweetened coconut: 131 calories

Nuts, one ounce serving:

- Slivered almonds: 170 calories
- Chopped peanuts: 166 calories
- Chopped walnuts: 184 calories

Cereals, one ounce serving:

- Cap'n Crunch: 114 calories
- Cinnamon Toast Crunch: 123 calories
- Froot Loops: 97 calories
- Granola: 138 calories

Cookies/Pretzels/Candy, one ounce serving:

- Oreo topping: 112 calories
- Crushed pretzel sticks: 110 calories
- Pretzels covered in chocolate swirl: 130 calories
- Milk chocolate M&Ms: 146 calories (1/4 cup has 210 calories)
- Gummi bears: 90 calories (14 pieces have 120 calories)
- Nestle crunch bar topping: 37 calories
- Heath bar, crumbled: 170 calories

24.

Some Questions To Ask Yourself When You're On The Brink Of Chowing Down

Your hand hovers over the food—your mouth is watering. What's triggering your "I really want to eat this" moment?

Eating triggers start a chain of events in motion, like overeating.

There are three general categories of triggers:

- Food
- Feelings
- The environment

Trigger Foods:

- are specific foods that start the type of overeating where you lose control and eat an excessive amount
- they're usually a combo of sugar and fat (brownies or gooey cookies)—or fat and salt (chips)
- they can be confused with your favorite foods (the ones that you really like), your comfort foods (ones that make you think of home, happiness, securtiy), or food cravings (when you want a food you haven't had in a while)

- it's the actual food not a feeling or place that triggers out of control eating

Trigger Feelings:

- are emotions, good or bad, that cause you to overeat (anxiety and sadness are common triggers)
- can prompt general out of control overeating—the kind where you shove large quantities in your mouth as quickly as possible

Trigger Environments:

- are specific situations or places that start a period of overeating (popcorn in a movie theater, going home for Thanksgiving)

What To Do

Before you eat it ask yourself:

- Is it fresh, tasty food? It might be if you're in your dining hall, it might not be if it's being handed out at the supermarket or sitting in a bowl on someone's desk.
- Is it clean? Think about this—how many fingers have been in the open bowl of peanuts or broken cookies?
- Do you really want it—or are you eating it just because it's there or because you're looking for comfort?
- Is it loaded with fat and sugar that add up to mega calories?
- If you fill up with non-nutritious junk food, will you skimp on good nutritious stuff later on because you're too full?
- If you eat it, will it open the floodgates so that you continue to indulge? Loading up on simple sugars—the kind in candy, cookies, cake, and many processed foods—will spike and then drop your blood sugar level and you'll be hungry and pretty darn cranky, too.

- If I really want to eat, can I find something that is better for me than junk food?
- If I remove myself from the place that I'm in, will my need/desire to eat go away?

25.

What Do You Eat With Your Movie?

What's the first thing you notice when you walk into the movie theater? Is it the wafting and delicious smell of freshly popped (perhaps not so freshly popped) popcorn?

It's no accident that the concession stand is placed right smack in the middle of the lobby. It sends your already conditioned eyes, nose, and salivary glands an urgent message: "Buy some"!

Even if you know that movie theater popcorn is a caloric nightmare, the siren call of freshly popped popcorn might be too strong to overcome.

I Don't Care, I'm Going To Have It Anyway

Even if you make it through the lobby without buckets or boxes in hand, all you have to do is sit down in the theater with someone near you noisily munching away. Up you go—back to the lobby and the concession stand where, thanks to slick marketing, you end up ordering the "bargain" combo: a jumbo popcorn and an extra large soda.

It's amazing what triggers us to eat. There's a research study by the Cornell food lab (eatouteatwell.com/bucket of popcorn) that shows that people overeat when they have large portions—even when they don't like the food. Moviegoers given stale popcorn in big buckets ate 34% more than people who were given the medium size of the same stale popcorn. People who had large buckets of fresh popcorn ate 45% more than people with the medium size.

What To Do

If you're going to eat in the theater, think about your choices.

- Would a small size of popcorn rather than jumbo do it for you?
- How about a regular candy bar instead of a king size or instead of one of those huge boxes of Goobers, Raisinets, or Milk Duds?
- If the popcorn, pretzels, or nachos look stale and nasty do you really want them?
- Ditch the soda for plain old water or a sugar free drink.
- You could bring some healthy snacks with you—like a lower calorie protein bar or trail mix (a crunchy apple doesn't lend itself to quiet eating).

Pretty Shocking Calories

Check the box or package for how many servings it contains. Movie theater boxes of candy are often huge and may be double or triple the size shown below. A large popcorn in one theater chain might be a medium in another. The number of cups of popcorn sounds crazy—but that's how much is in the common boxes or bags.

Popcorn, Nachos, Soft Pretzels

- Buttered popcorn, small, 5 cups: 470 calories, 35g fat
- Buttered popcorn, large, 20 cups: 1640 calories, 126g fat
- Cheese nachos, large, 4 ounces: 1100 calories, 60g fat
- Soft pretzel, large, 5 ounces: 480 calories, 5g fat

Soda and Lemonade

- Coke, 20 ounce bottle: 240 calories, 65g sugars
- Coke, small cup (18oz): 218 calories
- Coke, large cup (44oz): 534 calories
- Minute Maid Lemonade, 18 ounces: 248 calories
- Minute Maid Lemonade, 44 ounces: 605 calories
- Snapple Lemon Tea, 16 ounces: 150 calories, 36g sugars

Candy

- Junior Mints, 3 ounce box: 360 calories, 7g fat
- Sno Caps, 3.1 ounce box: 300 calories, 15g fat
- Milk Duds, 3 ounce box: 370 calories, 12g fat
- Raisinets, 3.5 ounce bag: 400 calories, 16g fat
- Goobers, 3.5 ounce box: 500 calories, 35g fat
- Twizzlers, 6 ounce bag: 570 calories, 4g fat
- M&Ms, 5.3 ounce bag: 750 calories, 32g fat
- Peanut M&Ms, 5.3 ounce bag: 790 calories, 40g fat
- Reese's Pieces, 8 ounce bag: 1160 calories, 60g fat

26.

Tired? Have Some Water

Dehydration causes fatigue. Even mild dehydration can slow your metabolism, drain your energy, and make you feel tired. Water is the main chemical component in your body and accounts for about 60% of your body weight. Every system in your body depends on it.

You need water for the chemical and metabolic processes to take place in your body; for body fluids like tears, sweat, and urine; to flush toxins out of your vital organs; and to carry nutrients to your cells.

There's no easy answer to the question: "How much water should I drink?" The answer really depends on many factors including your health, your age, how active you are, and where you live. For the average healthy adult who lives in a temperate climate, the Institute of Medicine recommends around 3 liters (about 13 cups) of total water intake a day for men and 2.2 liters (about 9 cups) of total water intake a day for women.

Total water intake includes drinking water, the water in beverages, and the water in food. All fluids count toward your daily total. On average, food supplies about 20% of total water intake. Many fruits and vegetables, like watermelon, grapes, lettuce, and tomatoes, are 90% or more water by weight. Food from grains like oatmeal and pasta are also hydrating because they swell up with water when they're cooked.

27.

Vending Machines: What's Your Favorite Letter/ Number Combination?

Sooner or later you will likely have your next sharing moment with a vending machine—you share your money and the machine shares its calories. It might happen on a road trip, game day, or in the middle of the night in your dorm.

Vending machines actually have a holy history. Around 215 BC the mathematician Hero invented a vending type device that accepted bronze coins to dispense holy water. Vending became economically viable In 1888 when the Adams Gum Company put machines on New York City elevated train platforms which dispensed Tutti-Frutti gum for a penny.

Now they're everywhere. They call your name when you're especially vulnerable—you're stressed, tired, bored, anxious, and your blood sugar is traveling south—all of which means the sugar, fat, and salt junk food allure is really hard to overcome.

No Choice Is Perfect; Make The Best Choice For You

With quarters or dollar bills in your hand, choose wisely. There are good, better, and best choices to be made. You can almost always find packages of nuts, popcorn, pretzels, or dried fruit along with the packaged sweet or crunchy calories.

Be careful of things with too much sugar, especially if you're driving. A big time sugar hit may give you quick energy but more than likely it will be followed by a drop in your blood sugar levels that could possibly make you sleepy, grouchy, unfocused, and hungry for more sweet and fatty food.

Your choice depends on what you want: protein or sweet satisfaction, fill-you-up fiber, or salty crunch. Here are some common choices.

Crunchy

- Baked! Lays Potato Chips (original), 1 package: 130 calories, 2g fat, 26g carbs, 2g Protein
- Baked Doritos, Nacho Cheese, 1 bag (38.9g): 170 calories, 5g fat, 29g carbs, 3g protein
- Cheez-It Baked Snack Crackers (Snack Pak): 180 calories, 9g fat, 20g carbs, 4g protein
- Ruffles Potato Chips, 1 package (1.5 ounces): 240 calories, 15g fat, 23g carbs, 3g protein
- Cheetos, Crunchy, snack size bag (1 ounces): 150 calories, 10g fat, 13g carbs, 2g protein
- Sun Chips Original, 1 package: 210 calories, 10g fat, 28g carbs, 3g protein
- Snyder's of Hanover Mini Pretzels, snack size: 160 calories, 0g fat, 35g carbs, 4g protein
- White Cheddar Cheese Popcorn, Smartfood, 1 package: 120 calories, 8g fat, 11g carbs, 2g protein

Nuts/Seeds

- Planters Sunflower Kernels, 1 package (1.75 ounces): 290 calories, 25g fat, 9g carbs, 11g protein
- Planters Salted Peanuts, 49g (1.75ounces): 290 calories, 25g fat, 8g carbs, 13g protein

Cookies/Pastry/Bars

- Mini Chips Ahoy!, snack pack (56g): 270 calories, 13g fat, 38g carbs, 3g protein
- Frosted Strawberry Pop-Tarts (2 pastries): 410 calories, 10g fat, 75g carbs, 4g protein
- Hostess Fruit Pie, apple: 470 calories, 20g fat, 70g carbs, 4g protein
- Fig Newtons, 1 package: 200 calories, 4g fat, 40g carbs, 2g protein
- Quaker Chewy Low-Fat Granola Bar, Chocolate Chunk, 1 bar: 90 calories, 2g fat, 19g carbs, 1g protein
- Nature Valley Granola Bar, Crunchy Oats and Honey, 2 bars: 190 calories, 6g fat, 29g carbs, 4g protein

Candy

- Skittles (original), 2.17 ounces: 240 calories, 2.5g fat, 56g carbs, 0g protein
- Twix, 2 cookies: 250 calories, 12g fat, 34g carbs, 2g protein
- 3 Musketeers, king size: 200 calories, 6g fat, 36g carbs, 1g protein
- Peanut M&Ms, 1 pack: 250 calories, 13g fat, 30g carbs, 5g protein
- Snickers, regular size: 250 calories, 12g fat, 33g carbs, 4g protein

28.

Eat More: Add In Healthy Foods To "Crowd Out" Less Healthy Food

There are fruit and veggies everywhere. Eat more of them. Eat more good food in general. But make it the healthy kind.

Instead of focusing on what you shouldn't eat and what you should take out of your diet, focus on what you can add in. Focus on adding in vegetables, fruit, and some whole grains.

When you load up on fruit, veggies, and whole intact grains that are rich in fiber and nutrients you help to displace—or "crowd out"—some of the foods in your diet that are higher in fat, sugar, and calories. And, as a bonus, you get the incredible benefits of all of the antioxidants and phytochemicals that are in the rainbow of produce that you're adding, plus the additional fiber to help keep you full.

What To Do

- If you fill your body with healthy, nutrient-dense food, you'll find that your cravings for unhealthy foods will naturally decrease.
- Try drinking a lot of water and eating nutrient dense whole food earlier in the day. It will help crowd out potential cravings later on in the day.
- Think outside the box, too. You don't have to focus on adding side dishes of vegetables or fruit salad for dessert. Add veggies

into your main dish—plump up burgers, meatloaf, or meatballs with chopped vegetables and/or some whole grains. Add cauliflower to mac and cheese. Mix fruit into your yogurt or cereal or use it as a topping for chicken or fish. Get creative!

29.

Home For Break: What Do You Grab To Eat When You're Stuck In An Airport Or A Train Station?

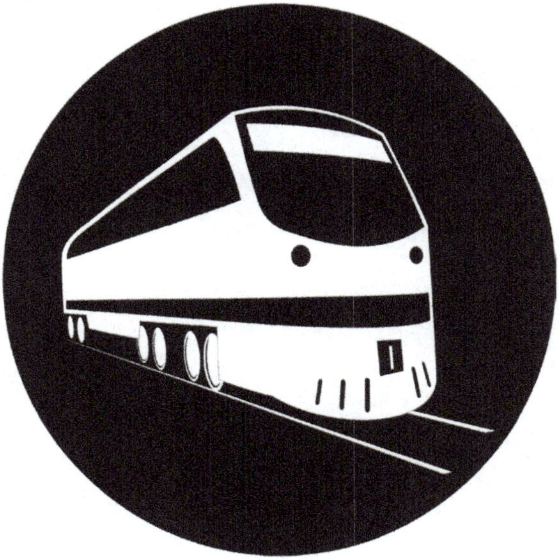

You get to the airport or train station, look up at the monitor, and see the dreaded words: delayed—or even worse: canceled. Canceled means scrambling and at least recognizing that you might need a real meal—delayed means being in limbo and not knowing what the heck to eat.

Then the meltdown: you might be hungry, maybe not. You're really annoyed because you have to hang around. You're going to be late for a connection, a reservation, getting home. You're angry and miserable. You hit the food stands.

Most larger airports and train terminals now have food courts with reasonably healthy food choices—if you choose to make them. But, if you're angry, tired, frustrated, what do most of us go for? Snack type food (read junk) and liquid calories.

Some Choices: Good And Not So Good

All packaged candy, chips, and bars have nutrition labels you can look at. Note that the serving and bag sizes for the foods listed below. The calories for snack and fun size candy aren't bad—multiply those figures for king size bars and large bags.

Snack Food

- Fritos, 28g, about 32 chips: 160 calories, 10g fat
- Ruffles potato chips, 28g, 12 chips: 160 calories, 10g fat
- Rold Gold Pretzel sticks, 28g, 48 pretzels: 100 calories, 0g fat
- Smartfood White Cheddar Popcorn, 28g, 1 ¾ cups: 160 calories, 10g fat
- Cracker Jack, 28g, ½ cup: 120 calories, 2g fat, 15g sugars
- Curly fries, 7 ounces: 620 calories, 30g fat
- Kettle corn, 31/2 cups: 245 calories, 6g fat
- Planter's Dry Roasted Peanuts, 1 ounce: 170 calories, 14g fat
- Blue Diamond Almonds, 1 ounce: 170 calories, 14g fat
- Planter's Nut & Chocolate Trail Mix, 1 ounce: 160 calories, 10g fat
- Beef Jerky, one large piece, 20g: 82 calories, 5g fat, 2g carbohydrate, 7g protein

Candy

- Raisinets, 1/4 cup: 190 calories, 8g fat
- Peanut M&Ms, about ¼ cup: 220 calories, 11g fat

- M&Ms, fun size bag: 73 calories; 3g fat
- Snickers, 1bar, 59g: 280 calories, 14g fat
- Large cotton candy: 170 calories, 0 fat
- Hershey's Milk Chocolate, snack size, 0.49 ounces: 67 calories; 4g fat
- Snickers, fun size: 80 calories; 4g fat
- Tootsie Rolls, 6 midgee pieces: 140 calories; 3g fat
- Skittles Original Bite Size Candies, fun size bag: 60 calories; 0.7 g fat
- Butterfinger, fun size: 85 calories; 3.5g fat
- Tootsie Roll Pop: 60 calories; 0g fat
- Starburst Original Fruit Chews, 2 pieces: 40 calories, 0.8g fat
- Brach's Candy Corn, 20 pieces: 150 calories, 0g fat
- Reese's Peanut Butter Cup, fun size: 80 calories, 4.5g fat
- Peppermint Pattie, fun size: 47 calories; 1g fat
- Kit Kat, fun size: 73 calories; 3.7g fat

Ice Cream

- Good Humor Chocolate Éclair, 1 bar, 59g: 160 calories, 8g fat, 11g sugars
- Fudgsicle Fudge Bar, 1 bar, 64g: 100 calories, 2.5g fat, 13g sugars
- Klondike The Original, 1 sandwich, 81g: 250 calories, 17g fat, 18g sugars

Water and Sports Drinks

- Gatorade: 12 ounces, 80 calories
- SoBe Lifewater: 20 ounces, 90 calories
- Glaceau Smart Water: 33.8 ounces, 0 calories
- Vitamin Water: 20 ounces, 125 calories
- Vitamin Water 10: 20 ounces, 25 calories

Coffee, Iced Coffee and Tea Drinks

- Dunkin' Donuts Vanilla Bean Coolatta, 16 ounces: 430 calories
- Dunkin' Donuts Sweet Tea, 16 ounces: 120 calories
- Starbuck's Coffee Frappuccino, 16 ounces (grande): 240 calories
- Starbuck's Coffee Frappuccino, light, 16 ounces grande): 110 calories
- Tazo Unsweetened Shaken Iced Passion Tea: 0 calories
- Iced Brewed Coffee with classic syrup, 12 ounces (tall): 60 calories
- Starbuck's Caffe Latte, 16 ounces (grande): 2% milk: 190 calories; 12g protein
- Starbuck's Cappuccino, 16 ounces (grande): 2% milk: 120 calories; 8g protein
- Dunkin' Donuts Vanilla Chai: 330 calories; 11g protein

Soda and Non-Carbonated Beverages

- Coke Classic, 20 ounce bottle: 233 calories
- Can of Coke, 12 ounces: 140 calories, 39g sugars
- Mountain Dew, 20 ounce bottle: 290 calories
- Snapple Orangeade, 16 ounces: 200 calories, 52g sugar
- San Pelligrino Limonata, 11.15 fluid ounce can: 141 calories
- Perrier Citron Lemon Lime, 22 ounce bottle: 0 calories
- Vitamin Water Focus Kiwi-Strawberry, 20 ounce bottle: 125 calories, 32.5g sugars
- Hint Blackberry, 16 ounce bottle: 0 calories
- Bottle of 7Up, 12 ounces: 150 calories, 38g sugars
- Gatorade G Orange, 12 ounce bottle: 80 calories, 21g sugars
- Coconut Water, 1 cup: 46 calories, 0g fat, 9g carbs, 2g protein
- Smoothie, Jamba Juice, fruit and veggie Tropical Harvest (original): 350 calories, 1g fat, 84g carbs, 3g protein
- Smoothie, Starbucks strawberry, 2% milk, 16 ounces: 300 calories, 2g fat, 60g carbs, 16g protein

30.

A Dozen Common Reasons We Eat When We're Not Hungry

Eating when you're not hungry, or when you're bored, angry, tired, procrastinating, or celebrating can push your calorie intake way up. The biggest problem is we often don't realize that we're shoving food into our mouths—either because we're distracted, we don't want to know, or we just plain old don't care.

What Makes Us Do It?

1. "Cheap" calories: the kind you find at all you can eat restaurants, freebie tastes in markets, "value and super sized meals."
2. Bread and extras like butter, olive oil, and olives on the table or peanuts or pretzels at a party. Way too tempting to pass up—especially if you're hungry or you've walked in with the attitude that you "deserve" it because you've had a tough day.
3. Opening the door to your room and having your favorite snacks staring you in the face (see it = eat it).
4. Procrastinating or avoiding doing what you have to do by having a snack.
5. Watching TV with a bag of chips or a bowl of candy on your lap.
6. Parties— especially when you drink—causing you to lose count and control of what you're grabbing to eat.

7. Dining halls that offer lots of food, lots of variety, and are open all the time.
8. High calorie food, freshly baked cookies, soda, beer, pizza, and lots of fried everything.
9. Care packages from home (either yours or your roommate's).
10. Feeling tired, stressed, overwhelmed, bored, angry, or "out-of-sorts" and turning to food as a "pick-me-up" or for comfort.
11. A big change in your exercise routine.
12. No one looking over your shoulder (like parents) to monitor what, when, and where you eat.

Bonus:

30 Quick Tips You Can Really Use

1. **Skip the bran muffin for breakfast.** We think bran muffins are "healthy" because they have the word bran in their name, but they're actually made with a lot of sugar and fat. A Dunkin' Donuts Honey Bran Raisin Muffin has 480 calories with 15 grams of fat and 79 grams of carbs (it does, however, have 5 grams of fiber). In general, a 4 ounce bran muffin has around 350 calories—but, have you seen the size of most muffins—they sure don't tip the scales at 4 ounces.

2. **A chocolate chip cookie—or oatmeal raisin for that matter—should be about the size of the rim of a soda can.** Some cookies are four times that size—and with four times the calories and fat content!

3. **Nuts are full of healthy fats and protein. They're a great snack and can help tide you over until your next meal—but they're also a high calorie food.** Be careful of portions—a serving size of most nuts is one ounce. For a one ounce serving:

    - 49 shelled nuts pistachios, 162 calories
    - 23 almonds, 169 calories
    - 21 hazelnuts, 183 calories
    - 18; cashews, 163 calories
    - 19 pecans, 201 calories
    - 14 English walnut halves, 185 calories
    - 10-12 macadamias, 203 calories
    - 39 peanuts (technically a legume),dry roasted, 170 calories

4. **Don't be duped by turkey, fish, and veggie burgers and sandwiches.** They sound healthier and less caloric than beef, but that might not be the case. At Red Robin a grilled turkey burger has 578 calories, 29g fat. Burger King's Premium Alaskan Fish sandwich has 530 calories, 28g fat while a Whopper Jr. without mayo has 260 calories, 10g fat. A Sedona Black Bean Burger at TGI Fridays has 870 calories, 49g fat.

5. **Bottled water isn't always just water.** Some are just water or water with flavor essence but lots of them are naturally or artificially sweetened, flavored, and colored. Don't be duped. For instance, many Vitaminwater flavors have 50 calories in a serving (8 ounces), but the bottles are usually 20 ounces which makes the contents around 120 calories and 30+ grams of sugar. There are no-calorie Vitaminwater Zeros, too.

6. **"Dilute" your pasta.** One cup of pasta has around 220 calories. Typical dinner portions can be as much as four cups. Increase the volume of what's on your plate by adding vegetables and decreasing the amount of pasta. Try adding mushrooms, cauliflower, broccoli, or eggplant. The calorie count will come down

(as long as the veggies aren't cooked with lots of oil), you'll have increased the nutrition of your dish, visually your portion will be substantial, and you'll feel quite full.

7. **Don't be sideswiped by smoothies.** They may be made with fruit and vegetables, but are often loaded with sugar. Unless you add a protein boost—a whey protein additive at Jamba Juice adds 45 calories and ten grams of protein—or your smoothie is made with yogurt or milk, they have hardly any protein. Jamba Juice's small (16 ounce) "Ideal Meal Chunky Strawberry" has 570 calories, 17 grams of fat and 54 grams of sugar. A small (16 ounce) healthy sounding "Berry Topper" has 480 calories, 9 grams of fat, and 55 grams of sugar. The original size Mango-A-Go-Go has 420 calories, 89 g sugar; the 16 ounce light version has 190 calories, 37g sugar.

8. **Cans and boxes that look like single servings may have two or three.** They may look small enough to be for one, but that doesn't mean it's true. Check out how many servings are in your can of soup or box of mac and cheese.

9. **If you have a sandwich for lunch—try these easy substitutions.** Use mustard instead of mayo and save 100 calories. Leave off the slice of Swiss cheese for another 133 calories. Ditch two slices of bacon for another 84 calories. Put your turkey, ham, or roast beef along with lettuce, tomato and onions in a whole grain pita (74 calories) instead of between two slices of rye (180 calories) and you've saved a total of 423 calories.

10. **Chinese food: even broccoli has calories.** If you think you're getting off easy because of all of the vegetables in Chinese food, think again. There are 466 calories in a cup and a half of beef and broccoli stir-fry (and about a day's worth of sodium). One cup of fried rice has 333 calories. If you include a vegetable spring roll for 63 calories and three fortune cookies for about 100 calories, your meal clocks in at around 1000 calories. Cut down a little bit, you probably won't even notice.

11. **Go for smalls and regulars**. Have a small cone instead of a 2 scoop, regular French fries instead of large, a small smoothie instead of a medium. Eat slowly and give your brain time to register the fact that you've fed your body some food. Don't fool yourself into thinking that a king size candy bar is a single serving. You'll probably be just as satisfied with the smaller portion and you'll have saved yourself a lot of calories.

12. **Leave the breadbasket at the other end of the table.** If you absolutely must have bread, go easy or without butter or oil. One teeny pat of butter has 36 calories, a tablespoon has 102 and 99% of them are from fat. A tablespoon of oil has about 120 calories

13. **Cut down on sugary drinks.** A 12 ounce soft drink has about 150 to 180 calories. A 16 ounce bottle of Snapple Orangeade has 200 calories; a 20 ounce bottle of Sobe Orange Carrot Elixir has 220 calories and a 12 ounce bottle of Ocean Spray Cranberry Juice cocktail has 180 calories. Substitute water for some or all of your daily drinks.

14. **Divide your food up into smaller portions and separate them to help avoid overeating.** Yale researchers took tubes of potato chips and made each seventh or fourteenth one red. The people who got to the red potato chip "stop signs" ate less than half as many chips than the people without the red chips and they more accurately estimated how much they'd eaten.

15. **Granola is a halo food—sounds like an angel but can be the devil in disguise.** Grains, oats and other ingredients are great—but not when they're mixed with too much sugar and fat. Look at the serving sizes, too—it could be a third of a cup. Who pours that into a cereal bowl? A quarter of a cup of Bear Naked's Fruit and Nut Granola has 140 calories, 7g fat. Kashi's GoLean Crunch has 200 calories, 3g fat in one cup.

16. **Avoid eating from a large open bag.** Count out your chips, crackers, and pretzels or only eat from a single portion size bag. Who can stop when there's an open bag of salty, crunchy food

right in front of you? It's amazingly easy to keep mindlessly eating until the bag is empty. A dive to the bottom of a 9 ounce bag of chips (without dip) is 1,260 calories. One serving, about 15 chips, is 140 calories.

17. **It's easy to be fooled by fatty sauces and dressings on innocent looking vegetables.** Vegetables are great. Veggies smothered with butter, cheese, croutons, and/or bacon are loaded with calories. Restaurants love to use oil and butter for flavor and to make the veggies glistening and mouth watering so they're often "rinsed" with oil just before they're served.

18. **Use a smaller plate.** We eat an average of 92% of what we serve ourselves. We pile more food onto larger plates (eatouteatwell.com/plate size), so a larger plate means we eat more food. A two inch difference in plate diameter—decreasing the plate size to ten inches from 12 inches—would mean a serving that has 22 percent fewer calories. It's a smaller serving but not small enough to leave you still hungry and heading back for seconds.

19. **Stop eating before you're full and keep away from seconds.** If you keep eating until your stomach finally feels full you'll likely end up feeling stuffed when you do stop eating. It takes a little time (around 20 minutes) for your brain to catch up and realize your stomach is full. A lot of eating is done with your eyes and your eyes love to tell you to try this and to try that. **Let this be your mantra: no seconds.** Choose your food, fill your plate, and that's it. Keep away from food spreads in the common room and open bags of anything to help limit nibbling and noshing.

20. **Use a fork and knife instead of your fingers, a teaspoon rather that a tablespoon.** Chopsticks slow you down even more. Chew your food instead of wolfing it down. If you have to work at eating your food—cutting with a knife for instance—you'll eat more mindfully than if you pick food up with your fingers and pop it into your mouth.

21. **Before you eat, drink some water, a no- or low-calorie beverage, or some clear soup.** The liquids fill up your stomach and leave less room for the high calorie stuff.

22. **Don't go to a party when you're starving**. How can you resist all the tempting food when your blood sugar is in the basement and your stomach is singing a chorus? Before you go eat a small healthy snack that's around 150 calories with some protein and fiber: fat free yogurt and fruit, a portion controlled serving of nuts, a small piece of cheese and fruit, or a spoonful of peanut butter with a couple of whole grain crackers. Have a calorie free or low calorie drink like water, tea, or coffee, too.

23. **Choose your food wisely.** If you can, pick lean proteins like fish, poultry, and the least fatty cuts of pork, beef, and lamb that are grilled or broiled, not fried or sautéed (look for the words loin or round, like tenderloin or eye round). Remember that beans and eggs are good sources of protein. Load up on vegetables—preferably ones that are not smothered in cheese or dripping with oil. Eat turkey without the skin.

24. **Don't eat all of the piecrust.** You can save around 200 calories at dessert by leaving the piecrust sitting on the plate and nixing (or decreasing) ice cream toppings like hot fudge sauce and whipped cream.

25. **Sprinkle bursts of activity through out your day.** These burn about 100 calories (150 pound person):

    - Pace when you're on the telephone instead of sitting
    - Run in place during television commercials
    - Swim laps at a moderate speed for 12 minutes
    - Casually bike for 23 minutes
    - Use the elliptical for 8 minutes
    - Walk stairs for 11 minutes
    - Do yoga for 20 minutes
    - Zumba for 11 minutes

- Do pilates for 24 minutes
- Dance around for 20 minutes
- Clean your room for 26 minutes
- Fly a kite for 20 minutes.
- Leisurely walk around campus for 51 minutes

26. **Before you grab some tasty morsel, ask yourself if you really want it.** Are you hungry? Is it worth the calories? Odds are, the tempting display of food in front of you is visually seductive—and may smell great, too—but you're reaching out to eat what's in front of you for reasons not dictated by your stomach but by your eyes. Have you decided that you want to splurge on something specific? Try picking it ahead of time and commit to your choice so you don't find yourself wavering in the face of temptation.

27. **Drink from a tall, thin glass instead of a short, wide one. You'll drink 25%-30% less.** People given short wide glasses poured 76% more than people who were given tall slender glasses, and they believed that they had poured less. Even experienced bartenders poured more into a short, wide glass.

28. **Is a half enough?** If you decide you really will feel totally deprived if you don't indulge in one of those delicious baked goods, choose one without loads of thick buttery crumbs on top, cut it in half or in thirds and be satisfied with that amount. Put it on a separate small plate that you can easily push away from you. Keeping it on your main plate or even a smaller one that's easily reachable means you'll be nibbling away at it the entire time.

29. Give yourself permission to eat—and enjoy—your favorite dessert or a burger or ribs. If you don't, you'll probably be miserable. Then when you get back to your room you end up gobbling down everything in sight because you made yourself miserable by not eating the stuff that you wanted in the first place! But no seconds and no first portions that are the equivalent of firsts, seconds and thirds built into one.

30. If you're full, stop eating and clear your plate right away. If it hangs around in front of you, you'll keep picking at it until there's nothing left. An exception—a study has found that looking at the "carnage"—the leftover bones from barbecued ribs or even the number of empty beer bottles—can serve as an "environmental cue" to stop eating.

You really are what you eat and drink. The effects of what you put into your body will show up now and years later, too. The choice is yours. You can still eat and drink great stuff; just control the not so great stuff—at least 80% of the time.

"You are what you eat"—is a shortened translation of the French phrase, "Dis-moi ce que tu manges, je te dirai ce que tu es" ("Tell me what you eat and I will tell you what you are"), which appears in (French physician) Anthelme Brillat-Savarin's book: "Physiologie du Gout, ou Meditations de Gastronomie Transcendante," 1826.

About The Author

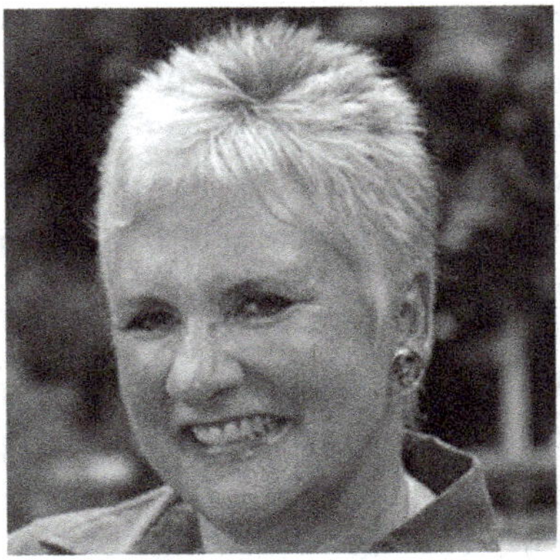

Penelope (Penny) Klatell, PhD, RN

Penny Klatell is a doctoral level nurse, a health and nutrition coach and a Mom. She's also a food lover, former college professor, author, blogger, speaker, and a very frequent restaurant visitor.

Penny grew up in the restaurant business. Her parents had an old fashioned New York City luncheonette—the kind with a long counter, booths in the back, a flat top grill, and a real malted machine. She learned about where food came from on her grandmother's working farm where all meals were made from scratch, eggs came from the chickens in the chicken coop, fruit came from trees and bushes, and vegetables came from the garden.

Penny raised three very active, athletic, and hungry sons who ate, studied, and played their way through college and graduate school and who taught her the meaning of having healthy and good tasting food available at all times – and in large quantities. Her family was—and is—a true proving ground for how to eat well . . . anytime, anywhere, and at any age.

Her books and blog, http://EatOutEatWell.com, include tips, strategies, and solid information about food, eating strategies, and weight management – all delivered with a bit of humor. She draws her information and inspiration from her love of food, visits to many restaurants and markets around the world, her professional and personal background, and a good deal of research drawn from trusted sources.

Her intent is to provide you with practical, usable information; help you love and learn about food; eat well; manage your weight; feed your family well; and bring a smile to your face.

Free gift for you!

As a bonus, go to:

http://EatOutEatWell.com/GetFoodMAP

and download your personal foodmap template to help you identify foods you love, your eating triggers, your eating pitfalls, and some good, better, and best eating strategies and choices.

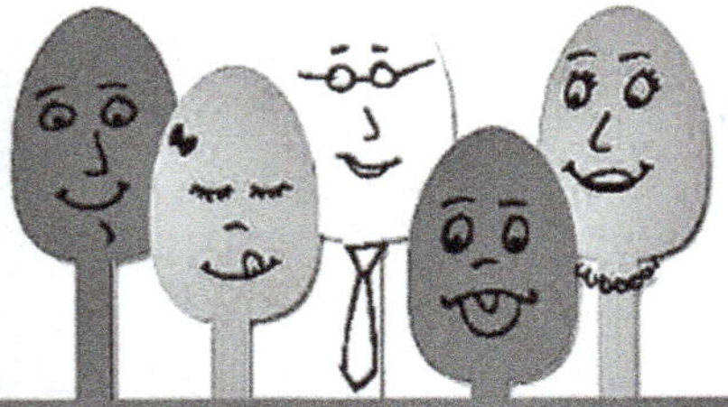

eat out
eat well
anytime, anywhere, at any age

Visit our blog at:

http://EatOutEatWell.com

Like & follow us:

Facebook.com/EatOutEatWell

Twitter.com/EatOutEatWell

Pinterest.com/EatOutEatWell

Google+ PenelopeKlatell

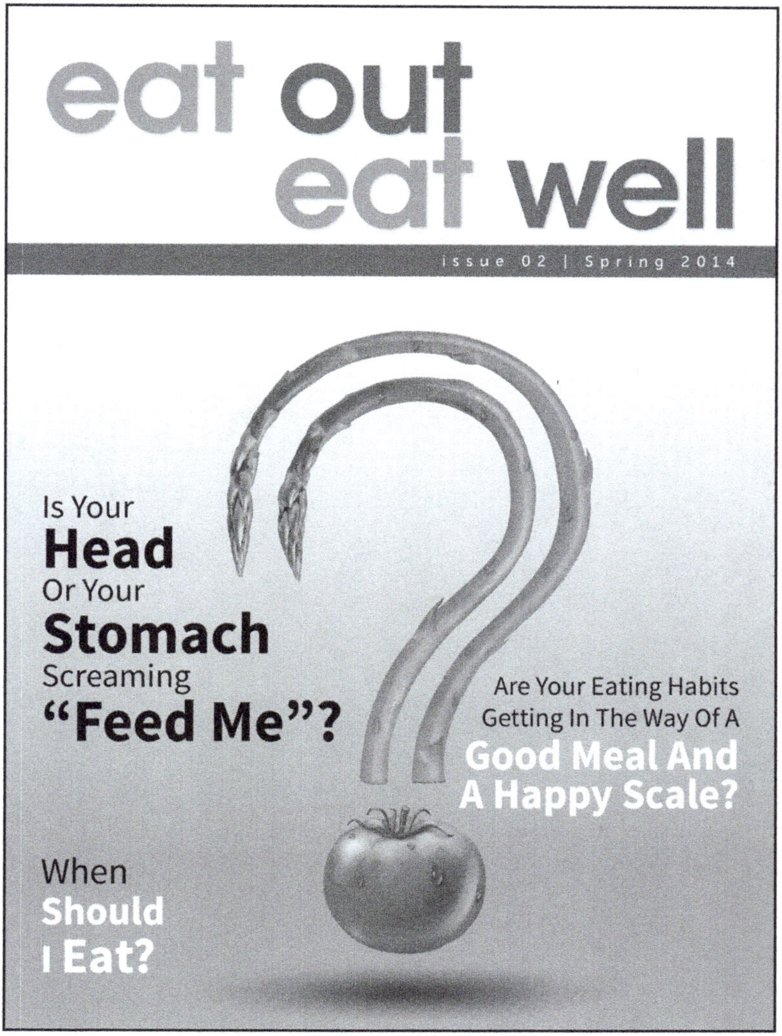

Visit Eat Out Eat Well Magazine, rated one of the top Health, Mind and Body apps on the newsstand in the iTunes store.

http://eatouteatwell.com/magazine

Made in the USA
Monee, IL
04 November 2026

67380106R00066

- Food is fuel for your body and brain. It can be both the culprit and the solution for a lack of energy, muddled thinking, and mid-afternoon drowsy eyes. But with an incredible amount and variety of dining hall food just begging to be heaped on your plate and no one looking over your shoulder, how do you make good choices?

- You've been eating everything in sight all day long -- capped by a 9PM trip to the vending machine. Why can you – and do you – still eat more even when you're stuffed?

- It's incredibly difficult not to eat gooey, salty, crunchy, and fatty foods when they're an integral part of campus life. How many times do your senses need to be assaulted by chips, wings, cookies, or some fried delight before you give in? What can you do?

- Alcohol doesn't fill you up the way food does because your GI tract and your brain don't register it as "food." But it does have calories—7 calories a gram—more than carbs and protein. So, you may not feel as though you're putting calories into your body, but you are.

Penelope (Penny) Klatell grew up in a restaurant family. She's a doctoral level nurse, a health and nutrition coach, and a Mom. She's also a food lover, former college professor, author, blogger at **EatOutEatWell.com**, a digital magazine editor, speaker, and a very frequent restaurant visitor.

Penny raised three active, athletic, and hungry sons who ate, studied, and played their way through college and graduate school and who taught her the meaning of having healthy and good tasting food available at all times – and in large quantities. Her family was—and is—a true proving ground for how to eat well … anytime, anywhere, and at any age.

my foodMAPs
YOUR ROADMAP TO HEALTHY EATING

ISBN-13: 978-0-9884767-3-8
(Ebook)

ISBN-13: 978-0-9884767-2-1
(Paperback)

Category: Health/Nutrition

ISBN 9780988476721
90000
9 780988 476721